THE OVER EASY
FOOT CARE BOOK

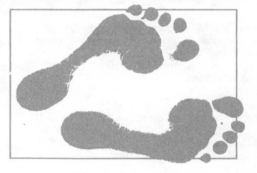

Timothy P. Shea, D.P.M.
Joan K. Smith

an AARP Book
published by
American Association of Retired Persons
Washington, D.C.

Scott, Foresman and Company
Lifelong Learning Division
Glenview, Illinois

DEDICATION

To my wife Amy and son Matthew for their
support and understanding. To Dr. George
Reiss and Dr. Philip Gardner for their
dedication and devotion to the care of the
aging human foot, and their ability to instill
this feeling in future doctors of podiatric
medicine.

T.P. Shea, D.P.M., F.A.C.F.O.

Copyright © 1984
Scott, Foresman and Company, Glenview, Illinois
American Association of Retired Persons, Washington, D.C.
All Rights Reserved
Printed in the United States of America
123456-KPF-888786858483

Library of Congress Cataloging in Publication Data

Shea, Timothy P.
  The over easy foot care book.

  Includes index.
  1. Foot—Care and hygiene. 2. Aging. I. Smith,
Joan K. II. Title.
RD563.S53 1984   617'.585   83-15881
ISBN 0-673-24807-0

PREFACE

THE OVER EASY FOOT CARE BOOK is a book about independence. Independence because if you've ever sprained your ankle or if your feet have ever hurt so badly you couldn't stand on them, you know what it means to *lose* your independence.

It's also about independence because it will introduce you to your feet and teach you to care for them as simply and inexpensively as possible. You can't treat every foot ailment yourself, but *you* are the primary care physician for your feet.

The first chapters deal with the relationship between foot health and general health. Chapters 4 through 8 discuss specific foot problems including symptoms, basic treatment and when to seek professional help.

Exercises, choosing footwear, and specific injuries are treated in Chapters 9 through 11. Chapter 12 discusses the benefits of walking and running, particularly in regard to the aging person. Surgery, medication, insurance, and alternative forms of treatment are dealt with in the final chapters. A glossary of terms explains words that may be unfamiliar to you.

By learning more about your feet, you will come to appreciate them more and take better care of them. In this way you may eliminate some minor problems and entirely avoid other foot problems in the future.

ACKNOWLEDGMENTS

Special thanks to those reviewers who carefully examined the manuscript and offered valuable advice:

Edward J. Busick, Jr., M.D., Joslin Diabetes Center, Boston, Massachusetts.

Louis G. Buttell, Public Affairs Director, American Podiatry Association, Washington, D.C.

Ron Hagen, Coordinator, AARP Insurance Services, Washington, D.C.

Norman Klombers, D.P.M., Executive Director, American Podiatry Association, Washington, D.C.

Chris McEntee, R.N., Health Care Specialist, AARP, Washington, D.C.

John McHugh, R.Ph., Director, AARP Pharmacy Service, Washington, D.C.

B. Alan Price, D.P.M., Lake Shore Foot Clinic, Chicago, Illinois; Munster Foot Clinic, Munster, Indiana.

Richard P. Reinherz, S.P.M., F.A.C.F.S., Editor of the *Journal of Foot Surgery*, Kenosha, Wisconsin.

Paul Spiegl, M.D., Special Fellow, Department of Orthopedics, Mayo Clinic, Rochester, Minnesota, 1982–83. Orthopedic Surgeon in private practice and Instructor, Grady Memorial Hospital, Atlanta, Georgia.

Nathan Zilber, R.Ph., Consultant, AARP Pharmacy Service, Washington, D.C.

TABLE OF CONTENTS

It's funny, you can always say that your foot hurts, and it sounds all right; but if you say that your feet hurt, it sounds perfectly lousy.
—Joan Crawford, as quoted in Reader's Digest,
September, 1936

Maybe you're exceptionally fond of your feet. You soak them, baby them, powder and paint them. You relish barefoot walks on sandy beaches and beg for foot massages. But most of us regard our feet with vague distaste, if we regard them at all, until they begin to hurt.

These mechanical wonders can break down. Foot problems are nearly as common as colds and headaches; four out of five adults experience them at one time or another.

Ironically, most foot problems are preceded by early symptoms we'd notice if we spent a few minutes a day checking our feet.

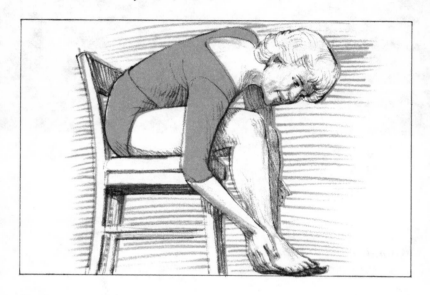

Inspecting your feet daily may alert you to small problems before they become more serious.

If you've ever had a foot problem or lived with some-one who has, you know that foot pain affects more than your foot. When you can't wear chic shoes or can't walk at all, your feet affect your social life, your ability to exercise and the way you generally feel.

But because pain is invisible, family and friends are sometimes unsympathic when severe foot pain interferes with your normal activities. People who have never had a foot problem often find it difficult to believe foot pain can be as disabling as it is.

Don't let others convince you the pain is in your head. Foot pain is very real and is usually caused by neglected feet, not by an overly active imagination.

FEET, WHAT GOOD ARE THEY?

By the time your're 55, you may have walked more than 70,000 miles, the equivalent of circling the globe two-and-a-half times. Each foot absorbs your weight with each step you take and two or three times your weight when you jog, run or dance.

Feet are also important to your circulatory system. Arteries that carry blood from the heart end in the foot. Working with the leg muscles to defy gravity, foot muscles pump blood back up through the veins in the legs to the chest cavity.

When your foot is too painful to move and you aren't using your foot muscles, the pumping action breaks down and fluid collects around your ankles and feet. The swelling, known as edema, indicates that your blood isn't circulating very efficiently to any part of your body.

YOU'VE GOT TO KEEP MOVING

It's difficult to over-emphasize the connection between walking and health. Psychiatrists commonly prescribe walking and even running to treat depression and, if you've had heart surgery, your doctor will almost certainly recommend that you begin to walk three to five miles a day as soon after the operation as possible. All the surgery in the world can't make up for inactivity's destructive effects on the heart.

Consider the difference between patients who enter convalescent homes and hospitals and remain physically and mentally active and those who give up their activities

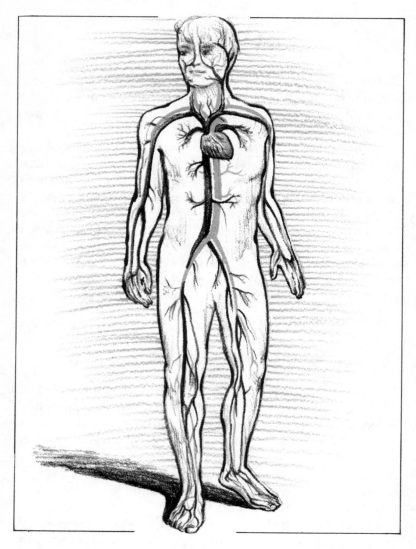

Feet are at the remote end of your circulatory system. They must work hard to pump blood back to the heart.

entirely. The former often recover and are released while those who give up often become completely disabled.

Exercise keeps the muscles, tendons and ligaments of the foot flexible, a flexibility feet need to adapt to the many kinds of shoes they wear and to the terrain they carry us over, be it a paved street or a beautiful dirt trail in the mountains.

Exercise keeps feet flexible, and flexible feet make it easier to keep exercising.

2

THE AGING FOOT

*Growing old isn't so bad
when you consider the alternative.*
—Maurice Chevalier

What does growing older mean to feet? They don't develop wrinkles or grow distinguished-looking, but they are affected by time.

Let's explore some of the changes you can expect to experience as your feet grow older and talk about how healthy feet can help the rest of you age better.

FLEXIBILITY

With age, your feet may lose a certain amount of flexibility.

Each foot is made up of 26 bones (a total of 52 for both feet or a quarter of all the bones in your body) plus 100

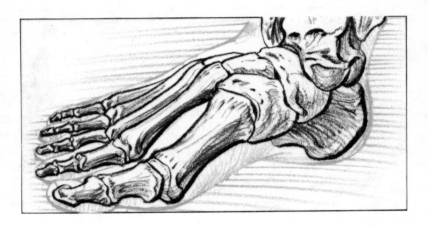

Each foot contains 26 bones. Together your two feet contain one-fourth of all the bones in your body.

small but important joints and miles of ligaments and tendons. When you're young, these joints and ligaments readily adapt to the shock of absorbing your weight with every step. As you grow older, structural changes like bunions and hammertoes can afflict these joints and limit their range of movement. At the same time, your ligaments and tendons are becoming less flexible and your foot needs more support and padding to adapt to the strain of carrying you around.

YOUR PRECIOUS FAT PADS

The bottom of every foot is lined with a protective, shock-absorbing cushion called a fat pad that helps protect fragile bones and joints from the impact of your feet hitting the ground.

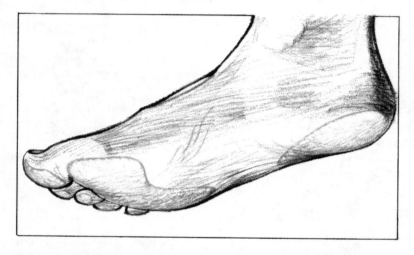

Fat pads on the bottoms of your feet protect bones and joints from the impact of walking.

Fat pads tend to thin out for several reasons. First, the constant trauma of walking in closed shoes on hard flat surfaces can push the fat pad, normally located in compartments on the bottom of the foot, up into other non-weight-bearing parts of the foot. In chronic hammertoes (bent toes), for instance, the fat pads are forced out from under the ball of the foot. The now unprotected, weight-bearing ball of the foot tends, as a result, to develop painful calluses.

Most of us consider smaller feet to be most attractive, so even if we do have thick feet, we tend to buy shoes that are too small and literally squeeze the protective padding out of its normal position.

Diabetes, arthritis and certain medications taken for high blood pressure can also cause thinning of the fat cells.

Changing nutritional needs is another reason fat pads often grow thinner with age. If you exercise and eat less as you grow older, your body tends to grow thinner, not only in your face, your neck and your upper body, but also in your feet. Your body draws upon its fat reserves for certain nutrients and tends to deplete any cushioning you might have.

Losing your foot's fat pad can be very painful. To have a very thin foot with no fat pad is to walk on skin and bones.

One indication of the fat pad's value is the extensive research that has been done on silicon and other fat-like materials that can be either implanted or injected into the bottom of the foot to form an artificial fat pad. Shoe inserts resilient enough to replace fat pads are also being studied.

WEAR AND TEAR

Years of walking affect not only bones, tendons and fat pads, they also take their toll on blood vessels and nerves.

With repeated trauma, a nerve running under the weight-bearing part of the foot can be trapped or pinched between skin and bone and grow swollen and painful. Eventually, a protective thickening called a *neuroma* or nerve entrapment grows around the nerve and becomes a constant irritant. Neuromas can be terribly painful. Victims describe sharp, stabbing sensations in the foot that often radiate to the toes or up the back of the leg.

Neuroma symptoms include pain and cramping in the ball and arch of the foot. Wearing shoes or walking often aggravates this condition. The pain and cramping is relieved to some extent by removing the shoes and either soaking or massaging the offending area. There are frequently nerve sensations, especially through the third and fourth toes, sometimes numbness and tingling, sometimes sharp, shooting pains. But the condition tends to persist and may become worse with time.

COLD FEET

Circulation commonly decreases with age and takes its toll on our feet.

Narrowed veins and arteries and subtler changes in the small blood vessels nourishing the skin and nerves of the feet can impair the foot's ability to adapt to the stress of walking and standing.

Conditions like diabetes can accelerate these changes, not only in the large blood vessels, but especially in the smaller vessels that nourish all soft tissues.

Impaired circulation literally starves the foot of nutrients, may eventually impair flexibility and may cause fluid retention and swelling in both the legs and feet. Since the foot is farthest from the heart, it is the first part of the body to be affected by decreased circulation.

Pay attention to changes in your feet. Puffy toes might be more serious than just a local foot problem. Avoid using garters, garter belts or stretch hose, all of which tend to constrict circulation.

ARTHRITIS

The word *arthritis* is from the Greek *arthron* meaning *joint* and *itis* meaning *inflammation* or *swelling*. The word suggests swelling of the joints.

Since arthritis affects the joints, the large network of bones in the feet is particularly vulnerable.

There are many types of arthritis. Three common types are gout, rheumatoid arthritis, and osteoarthritis. Gout is a buildup of uric acid crystals. It results from abnormal breakdown of food products in the system. Although these crystals can collect in the ear lobes, elbows, knees and wrists, they settle most commonly around the ankle and bones of the foot, especially the big toe joint. The foot becomes inflamed, stiff, and can be very painful. This condition is called "podagra."

Rheumatoid arthritis is a deforming metabolic condition that afflicts victims of every age. With no known cause, acute rheumatoid arthritis attacks only at intervals, but it's always present in a latent state. It strikes women more often than men and can cause severe permanent damage especially in children. If severe, rheumatoid arthritis can be a crippler.

But the one form of athritis directly associated with age is osteoarthritis. Osteoarthritis or wear-and-tear arthritis is the erosion of cartilage around the joints and the natural degeneration of joints, bones and tendons that comes with years of use and abuse.

Wear-and-tear arthritis can begin to affect you in your twenties. On the other hand, you might never notice it. Its most common effect is a certain amount of discomfort and limited flexibility. Joints tend to become stiff and painful and always become deformed.

BACK PAIN AND YOUR FEET

There's probably nothing more disabling than back pain but very few people realize that a fair percentage of back problems are literally rooted in foot problems. Back problems may also cause foot problems that in turn reinforce the back problem. This is true of conditions ranging from simple nervous tension in the shoulders and neck to abnormal curvatures of the spine.

Back problems are related to feet because it's the foot's job to absorb the stress of movement, to adapt to the terrain, to function in shoes and to compensate for any weaknesses in the spine. Though it probably doesn't make sense to treat a spinal condition without considering the foot, many doctors don't include a foot exam in the evaluation of a back problem.

Whether the treatment for back pain is a muscle relaxant, a back brace, physical therapy or massage and spinal manipulation by an osteopath or chiropractor, the results won't be permanent unless any corresponding imbalance in the foot is corrected.

No single part of your body can be effectively repaired in isolation. People who complain of foot fatigue or arch fatigue or who wear out shoes in a certain pattern usually have back pain. When you seek treatment for back pain, be sure to have your feet evaluated, too.

SHOES

From the time you're a toddler and are fitted for your first pair, shoes affect the way your feet develop. Although they aren't the only cause of foot problems, shoes can aggravate existing conditions so that minor problems often become disabling with age.

Comfortable shoes can prevent pain from corns, calluses, bunions and other foot problems. Shoes are more important now than they ever were because paved streets and sidewalks have dramatically added to the stress our feet absorb.

Finding comfortable shoes isn't easy, though. Orthopedic shoes, for instance, are not stylish. We picture them as black shoes with laces and two-and-a-half-inch heels. These aren't orthopedic shoes, even if they have arch supports.

A true orthopedic shoe is molded to the foot, has only enough heel height to provide support and has lots of room for your toes. When older feet become less resilient, they need shoes that will absorb some of the shock to which they're no longer able to adapt.

The outer sole should be firm but spongey enough to absorb the shock of walking. New space-age materials with these attributes are replacing the familiar leather and rubber soles. The upper portion of the shoe should conform to the foot and not be constricting in any way. The heel counter should fit the back of the heel. The ball of the foot should fit comfortably in the shoe.

But buying molded, orthopedic shoes is a difficult decision to make. They're fairly expensive and are never modeled in the pages of the fashion magazines. Most of us still buy fashion over function, no matter what the cost.

MOBILITY FOR A HEALTHIER, LONGER LIFE

Your vitality is directly related to your ability to move. Too many people in their seventies and eighties lose their enthusiasm for life when they can't get around.

Exercise is one of the best ways to prevent serious illnesses we tend to develop when we're older. Exercise can help control high blood pressure, relieve arthritis symptoms, and improve your mood.

Exercise is also one of the most important aids to recovering from any kind of surgery. When you're confined to a bed or chair for any length of time, you lose a certain amount of endurance. It can take a week or two to get back into shape even if you've only been laid up for a few days.

More people are hospitalized and operated on in the United States than anywhere else in the world, but until recently, not much attention was paid to caring for the hospitalized patient's feet. Today, most hospitals have podiatrists who can care for acute or disabling foot problems and help patients regain mobility after their hospital visit.

There was a young lady of Crete
Who was so exceedingly neat,
When she got out of bed
She stood on her head
To make sure of not soiling her feet.
—Bennett Cerf's Out on a Limerick

If your feet could talk they'd probably conspire to revolt. Fortunately, they can't discuss the hard work and neglect they endure, but they can complain to you in the language of pain. We refer to bunions, hammertoes, ingrown toenails and corns as common foot problems. But they're not just problems; they're the vocabulary of unhappy feet. You can prevent foot problems with regular care.

A SIMPLE DAILY ROUTINE

Bathe your feet daily in a pan of lukewarm (not hot) water using a mild face soap. Work up a lather and scrub lightly in and around your toenails and between your toes. Gently rub a pumice stone, callus file, or special abrasive sponge on rough or thickened skin that accumulates on your heels and the bottoms of your feet (unless you have circulation problems or sensitive skin). First soak your feet to moisten and soften those areas.

Dry your feet thoroughly, especially between your toes. Sprinkle them with a foot powder that does not contain starch or moisturize them with a soft lotion or cream. Avoid using lanolin and alcohol.

Clip your toenails straight across with a clipper designed for toenails. Nails should be trimmed so that you can see the leading edge all the way across.

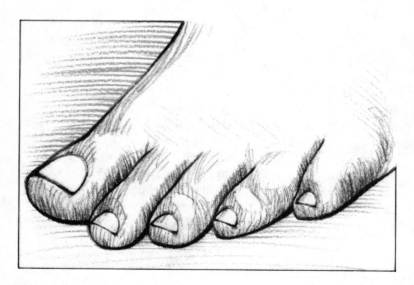

Trim your toenails straight. The toenail should extend beyond the toe all the way across.

Check your feet daily for cracks or redness. If skin is cracked you should see your doctor. Dry skin is an excellent breeding ground for bacteria and fungi. A moisturizing cream will help. Most lanolin-based creams are okay, but don't use petroleum-based products because they don't let feet breathe. Don't use alcohol-based products because they can cause drying. In addition, these products aren't easily absorbed into the skin and can make your feet slide around in your socks and shoes.

Rest your feet whenever you have a few moments to yourself. Elevate them above heart level to relieve pressure.

Massage your feet to maintain flexibility and relieve tension. Start the massage at the ball of the foot, kneading with your fingertips. Work along the sole to the heel. Push each toe back and forth gently to relax and relieve tired, tense muscles.

Do some of the exercises described in Chapter 13.

A WARNING

Don't try to doctor your own feet:
- If you're diabetic,
- If you have severe circulatory problems,
- If you've developed an infection,
- If you have severe allergies and are sensitive to over-the-counter medicines,
- If you can't see well,
- If your hands are unsteady for any reason,
- If you have arthritis affecting your hips, knees or spine that makes it painful to reach your feet,
- If a problem remains for any period of time or if a problem regularly reoccurs.

HOW TO FIND A DOCTOR

This is a difficult question and one that's never answered in a satisfying way.

If you already have a family doctor you trust, you're in good shape. He or she may not be willing or able to treat your foot problem but will refer you to a podiatrist or another specialist who can.

If you don't have a doctor, ask friends and acquaintances whose judgment you trust to recommend one. Don't settle for names; find out why they like their doctor. You might have different criteria.

You can also get a referral from the American Podiatric Association or from your local American Medical Association. Podiatrists are the only doctors who specialize in foot care. They go to podiatry schools and are called doctors of podiatric medicine (DPM) rather than medical doctors (MD).

If you have a severe bunion or another structural problem that might require surgery, your doctor might refer you to either a podiatrist or to an orthopedic surgeon. Orthopedic surgeons specialize in surgical correction of skeletal deformities.

Most medical practitioners agree that it is best to have a family doctor who knows you and your history and who can refer you to a specialist as necessary.

NAIL PROBLEMS

4

Why doesn't medical science find some
way to make our ailments as interesting
to others as they are to us?
—Harold Coffin

Nails may not be the mirrors of the soul, but they are excellent indicators of your overall medical condition. Toenails often show the first signs of serious disorders like diabetes, infections, drug reactions, and poor nutrition. Pitting and excessive ridging of the nail might indicate insufficient circulation, for instance.

As you grow older, your toenails are the one part of your foot most vulnerable to painful problems. Every day they are repeatedly compressed by tight hosiery and jammed into the front of your shoe as you walk. The accumulation of these small traumas can eventually produce an injury every bit as serious as an injury caused by dropping a five-pound parcel on your toe.

Doctors usually categorize nail problems by the nail's appearance. There are ingrown nails, thickened nails, and thinning nails, all of which sometimes result in loss of the entire nail.

INCURVING AND INGROWN NAILS

Ingrown nails or nails that begin to cut or grow into the skin are the most common foot problem among older people. They can be caused by tight shoes, but usually ingrown nails are caused by improper nail trimming. Most people get carried away with their nail clippers and cut away too much of the nail. Ingrown toenail occurs most often in the large toe but other toes can also be afflicted. Sometimes ingrown toenails are so painful you can't wear shoes.

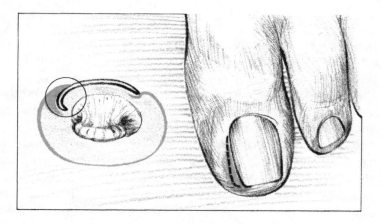

Ingrown toenails often result from improper trimming. They can be very painful. Left illustration shows ingrown toenail as seen from the front of the toe.

Untreated, an ingrown nail can break through the skin leaving your toe vulnerable to infection. Any infection should be treated by a podiatrist immediately because infections can spread into the rest of the body. Left untreated, ingrown toenails also can cause the tissue around the nail to thicken and become painful.

Don't mistake an incurving or C-shaped nail for an ingrown one. C-shaped nails seem to curve directly into the skin. They occur when the nail matrix or root is deformed. The nail bed thickens and a distorted nail begins to develop. When incurving nails aren't trimmed properly, they can become ingrown. If you have a C-shaped nail, don't try to trim or treat it until you've consulted your doctor.

THICKENED NAILS (HYPERTROPHY)

The most common thickened nail is due to fungus. A chronic fungus, similar to athlete's foot, grows up under the nail and, when the front edge of the nail is lifted by the normal trauma of walking in shoes, the fungus creeps into the nail and grows uninhibited.

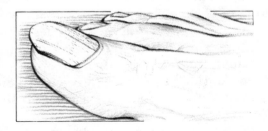

Fungus can cause a thickening of the toenail. It can damage the nail plate and the nail matrix and is difficult to treat.

Nail discoloration is an early sign of fungus infection. Yellow, white or brownish streaks appear along the edges of the nail and sometimes run down the middle. They grow more pronounced with time.

As the fungus grows further under the nail, it grows into the matrix tissue and actually lifts the nail up from its attachment to the skin. The fungus tissue starts to replace the nail, which has begun to grow away from the toe bed, and the nail becomes brittle. If the fungus is allowed to grow into the closed end of the nail around the cuticle, the entire nail will become thick, yellowish, chalky and very brittle.

Fungus nail usually forms a bulge on the top of the toe and makes it painful to wear shoes. At a certain point, it begins to affect the cells that produce the nail creating odd deformities; the nail might begin to grow sideways or loop back toward the toe.

None of this happens overnight. Fungus nail is a chronic, insidious process and the changes it causes usually occur over a long time.

It's difficult to eradicate the fungus that causes this nail problem because no over-the-counter medicine can penetrate the thickened nail to reach the fungus. It's also difficult to trim these nails because they tend to crumble and break off in pieces leaving ragged edges behind.

After you've trimmed and scrubbed the nail, apply an over-the-counter antiseptic like tincture of iodine or gentian violet solution once or twice a week. If you do this regularly, a normal nail should appear within six months to two years.

This treatment can dry out the skin around the nail. If you notice drying, cracking or bleeding, discontinue treatment until the skin is normal again. And if you have to discontinue treatment for this reason, if the nail doesn't respond, or if the nail grows thicker and begins to crack and put pressure on the toe, see your doctor.

Professional treatment of fungus nail generally involves applying medicine to the nail that will dissolve both the nail and the fungus under it. Oral medication is sometimes prescribed. Medication is usually repeated until a new nail grows in.

If the condition is longstanding and has progressed deeply under the nail, a podiatrist can surgically remove the nail and apply medicine to destroy the cells that produced the nail.

Fungus nail can be a sign of serious illness. One form, a yeast infection that commonly appears as a white discoloration of the nail and an accumulation of white tissue between the toes, is an early sign of diabetes.

Fungus is everywhere. It's in the air, in the soil, in our shoes, in the showers. It's impossible to completely sterilize our environment to free it of fungus. The best prevention of fungus nail is good foot hygiene consisting of bathing your feet daily, keeping nails properly trimmed and avoiding shoes and socks that irritate your nails. Use a mild soap, and sprinkle powder inside your shoes. Disinfect your shoes with ultraviolet light or direct sunlight. Most important, be sure to wear *dry* shoes and socks. Natural blend, cotton and wool socks and natural leather shoes are better than synthetics.

INJURED NAILS

Nail traumas range from the relatively minor but constant irritation of tight shoes, high-heels or a thickened nail to the impact of something heavy falling directly on your foot. A forceful blow to the nail will usually produce a hematoma or blood-blister under the nail. A hematoma is initially very painful and eventually the nail may fall off. Cool soaks will usually reduce the swelling and discomfort. If soaks don't relieve the pain or if there is active bleeding, you should seek professional care.

NAIL CARE

A regular nail hygiene program can prevent nail problems. It should include trimming your nails every four to six weeks as necessary. Nails should be clipped straight across just slightly longer than the end of the nail lip on each side of the nail. If the sides of the nails tend to curve in, trim them very gently and file away any rough edges at the corners with an emery board or consider packing with a small amount of cotton.

Soaking your feet in warm, soapy water for five to ten minutes before trimming your nails will soften and make them easier to trim. If the area around your nails is sore, seek professional advice.

Wear shoes and socks that fit you. Tight footwear will irritate the nail and make your toe feel as if the nail is ingrown whether it is or not.

SKIN PROBLEMS

5

And when too short the modish shoes are worn,
You'll judge the seasons by your shooting corn.
—John Gay, Trivia Bk. i, l. 33

Like bones and joints, skin tends to lose elasticity with age. Skin without the resilience to absorb friction is vulnerable to corns, calluses and more serious problems like ulcers and infections.

If your circulation is poor, your skin is probably shiny and dry and vulnerable to cracking and injuries. Regular use of an emollient or lanolin-based lotion or ointment will keep your skin moist.

You'll probably also see more pigmented spots as you grow older. Though these are rarely malignant, they should, like any new growth or changing lesion, be investigated by a doctor.

Skin irritations like corns, calluses and ulcers are often aggravated by ill-fitting shoes, but they are often caused by a deformity or functional imbalance in your feet or legs.

CORNS

Corns afflict people of all ages, generally on a toe which tends to rub against a shoe or a toe that is out of line with the others.

Repeated friction irritates the toe and increases the blood supply which in turn accelerates cell production of cornified substance. The corn develops to protect the area. The hard central core of the corn kills the cells below in a cone shape over the point of bone pressure or shoe irritation. The deeper the corn grows, the more likely its pointed end will irritate a nerve if any external pressure is applied to it.

A fluid-filled sac or bursa overlays and protects each joint in your body. If the core of a corn presses against a toe joint, it can irritate the bursa. Too much irritation causes bursitis, a painful swollen bursa.

You can treat a mildly irritating corn at home. First find out the cause and eliminate that. Often the cause is ill-fitting shoes or hosiery. If changing footwear doesn't help, cut a piece of plain moleskin into thin strips and place them on your afflicted toes to reduce friction between the toes and your shoes. Either get your shoes stretched or buy shoes with a wider toe box to prevent further irritation.

You should also soak your toes daily in warm soapy water and apply a softening cream. Then scrub the corn with a pumice stone or emery board to keep the skin from thickening.

Use over-the-counter corn removers with caution. They are caustic and cause severe burns. Never do bathroom surgery; it's too easy to cut normal tissue when you use razor blades or scissors to trim hard tissue. Such cuts are easily infected or can also result in painful scar tissue.

Corns tend to reappear. If caring for them at home doesn't seem to be effective, consult your podiatrist to determine the best appropriate treatment.

SOFT CORNS

Soft corns usually appear between the fourth and fifth toes. They result from pressure of bony protuberances on neighboring toes or of poor alignment.

The moisture between your toes keeps the corn soft.

Soft corns usually develop more slowly than hard corns and they're often mistaken for fungus infections. Untreated, soft corns can become painful fissures, deep splits in the skin that leave the foot vulnerable to infection.

Fissures are usually very painful and require professional care consisting of antiseptic soaks and padding between the toes.

To ease the pain of soft corns, use lamb's wool to separate your toes. Wrap the strands in loose, thin layers around the afflicted toes to relieve pressure. Use powder to keep the area dry and wear cotton socks or stockings that will absorb perspiration.

If soft corns are a chronic problem for you, see your doctor. Sometimes minor surgery to remove the irritating bony prominence is necessary.

PLANTAR CALLUSES

Plantar refers to the bottom of your foot, so plantar calluses are simply calluses that develop on the bottom of your feet.

Like corns, calluses develop to protect the foot against excess friction, but over a wider area.

Calluses appear naturally to protect the feet of people who frequently walk barefoot on rough surfaces, but if calluses develop while you're wearing shoes, they're probably a sign of some structural imbalance.

Calluses often indicate incorrect weight distribution. High-heeled shoes, for instance, put all the weight on the ball of the foot and tend to cause large calluses in that area.

Calluses consist of keratin (a cell secretion) and they aren't in themselves painful. So when a callus does hurt, it's probably putting pressure on the nerve and blood vessels beneath it.

Simple callus care consists of soaking your feet for 15 minutes in warm water and applying a moisturizer two or three times a day. Once calluses are softened, rub them gently with a pumice stone or another mild abrasive. Performing this ritual three nights in a row should soften even the toughest callus. Making it a part of your routine—two or three nights a week—will soothe your feet and keep them soft.

CENTRAL CORE CALLUS

Besides the generally thickened tissue of the normal callus, some calluses form a rock-hard center at the weight-bearing part of the foot. This core is dead tissue that grows into the sweat ducts on the bottom of the foot.

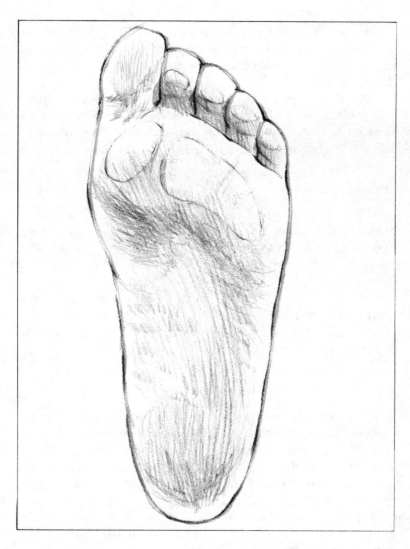

Plantar calluses are those that develop on the bottom of the foot.

Core calluses are extremely painful and don't respond well to simple soaks and padding. They are sometimes mistaken for warts, but warts are relatively uncommon in the aging foot.

Core calluses require professional treatment. Usually only a bit of medication applied to the area will reduce the swelling of the core but sometimes the core must be surgically removed.

CALLUS COMPLICATIONS

Like a corn, an untreated plantar callus can irritate a bursal sac overlaying the joints and result in bursitis. Bursitis is painful, but it can be excruciating if the swollen bursa breaks and traps a nerve under the skin forming a neuroma.

Your doctor can treat bursitis with anesthetics and mild anti-inflammatory steroids. In some cases, it's necessary to have the trapped nerve or bursal sac removed in order to relieve the painful inflammation.

FOREIGN BODIES

When a splinter, bit of glass or another foreign object is embedded in your foot, your body forms a wall of tissue around it to protect the rest of you from the invasion. If you didn't feel the invasion in the first place, you probably won't understand the cause of the red, painful swelling on the bottom of your foot. Eventually the area may open up in a pustule (pustules are filled with pus). Sometimes you'll find the foreign body in the middle of these when they break. Otherwise the protective tissue thickens around the splinter forming a hard core surrounded by a spreading callus.

A good precaution is to check your feet and footwear (shoes and socks) daily for embedded bits of matter, especially if you're a diabetic. If you find a splinter or bit of glass, soak your feet twice a day in warm (not hot) water. Adding three tablespoons of Epsom salts to a quart of water will help draw the material to the surface. Seek professional advice. This could be a very dangerous condition.

After your soak, clean the affected area with rubbing alcohol, pat it dry and inspect it for debris. The soaks should help remove foreign bodies and within two or three days the pain and swelling should disappear. If they don't, see your doctor.

Remember that if you're a diabetic or have another severe circulatory problem, you should never try to treat yourself. Your doctor will probably anesthetize the painful area and remove the foreign matter with any hard thickened skin around it.

If you walk around at night, be sure to wear slippers. Many people, when they wander around barefoot in the dark, seem to pick up these foreign particles.

ULCERS

Poor circulation affects your skin. It causes hair loss, discoloration, skin that feels cool to the touch and skin that is especially vulnerable to ulcers.

Stasis ulcers are the most common. They usually afflict skin in the ankle areas, the heels and the sides of the foot and often accompany phlebitis and varicose veins. If you're partially bedridden, you might also develop them from your ankles pressing against the sheets and from constant pressure and inactivity.

Stasis ulcers first appear as itching and/or redness around the bony prominences of the ankle and foot. Scratching irritates the skin which, having lost its elasticity, begins to peel. The resulting ulcer is a draining, painful, infected wound along the inner or outer side of the leg and, if left untreated, can spread and infect the bone.

Stasis ulcers are caused by blood pooling in the tissues when the muscles in the leg are unable to pump blood toward the heart. Therefore the object in treating stasis ulcers is to move the blood out of the tissue.

If your doctor has advised you to treat stasis ulcers at home, elevate your foot on two pillows, clean the wound with hydrogen peroxide and dry bandages, and apply a sterile non-stick gauze pad with an elastic bandage. Do this two or three times daily. When the ulcer has healed, you can prevent a new flare-up by wearing support hose and doing foot exercises to improve circulation. (See Chapter 13 on Exercise.)

If an infection is present you'll need to seek professional help before it spreads. In the early stages, your doctor or podiatrist may prescribe a compressive dressing, treat the infection, and prescribe special shoes, support hose, or exercises for the feet and legs to improve circulation. When necessary, the podiatrist will refer you to a peripheral vascular surgeon.

Diabetic ulcers often appear on the bottom of the foot, usually around the ball of the foot, on the outside arch or around the heel. These ulcers often don't hurt because diabetics have very little feeling in their feet. A diabetic ulcer is dangerous because the high carbohydrate sugar concentration in the skin and lack of circulation make the skin a perfect medium for bacteria. Diabetic ulcers should always be treated by a doctor.

Bedsores are ulcers that usually occur on the heel or ankle or on the outside of the foot. When you're confined to your bed, inactivity tends to diminish circulation. Your skin loses nourishment, breaks down and is susceptible to ulcers. You can't leave the source of the problem—your bed—but you can prevent bedsores. Use lambswool heel and foot protectors to protect yourself from abrasion. Foam rubber ankle and heel elevators will keep your feet and legs off the bed. To balance the stress on your feet, you should also avoid lying constantly on one side.

6

STRUCTURAL PROBLEMS

If you chew well with your teeth,
you'll feel it in your toes.
—Talmud

BUNIONS

Though most of the aging foot's problems are skin-related or nail-related, many are caused by changes in the bones and joints.

A bunion, for example, is the swelling of the bursa (protective fluid-filled sac) overlaying the big toe joint. It's caused by a disorder called *hallux abducto valgus* (*hallux* means *great toe, abducto* means *outward, valgus* means *rotation*), in which the big toe turns toward the other toes and its joint protrudes from the side of the foot. The friction between the protruding joint and your shoes causes the swollen bursa and joint capsule.

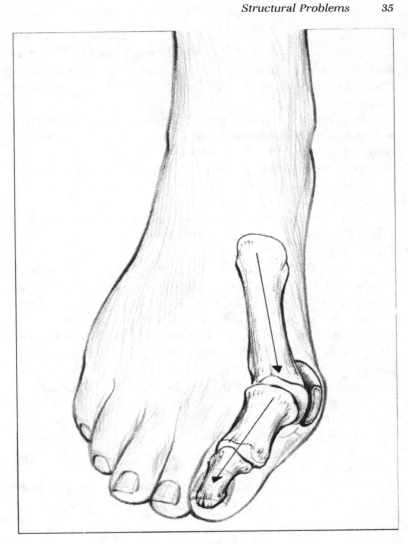

A bunion occurs when a bursa over a joint is irritated and begins to swell.

Bunions frequently are hereditary. However, inflammatory diseases like gout and rheumatoid arthritis can break down joints, too, and allow the angle of the big toe to increase.

Bunions are not only unsightly; frequently they can be very painful. As bunions progress, internal joint arthritis may develop. When you adapt to a bunion, it usually becomes less swollen and painful but this is no guarantee that the intense pain won't flare up again as the bunion deformity increases.

Because bunions are rooted in a structural or functional problem, they're most effectively helped by diagnosing the cause and correcting that.

Short of surgery, you might find relief by treating it yourself. Foot soaks are soothing and can temporarily relieve swelling and pain. Over-the-counter pads and toe separators produced for bunions can cushion them against further irritation. Sometimes a combination-last shoe—with a size A heel and a size C toe, for instance— can provide relief, especially if it's fitted with a special pad to cushion the bunion. Molded shoes, built to conform to the shape of your feet, may offer some help in relieving pain of bunions.

Bunion surgery sometimes may be done on an outpatient basis under a local anesthetic and you can walk out after the operation. If, like most of us, you're afraid to have surgery, discuss your concerns with your doctor. You may also want to get a second opinion before surgery.

HAMMERTOES

A hammertoe looks like a little hammer in a piano. The tendons and ligaments hold the toe up and back so it's in a

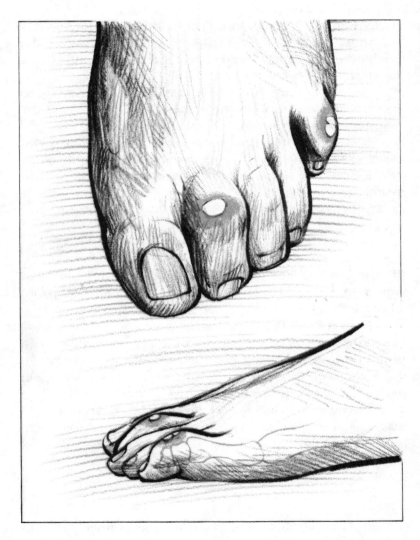

Hammertoes are permanently bent up and back. They may become more rigid and develop painful corns with time.

permanently bent position. Feet with high or low arches are most likely to develop hammertoes because of the positioning of the ligaments and tendons. The fifth toe is most often the victim.

Tight shoes and high-heels are extremely irritating to hammertoes. Sometimes they cause them by forcing the ligaments into unnatural positions.

With age, hammertoes may become more rigid and develop painful corns. In this case, surgery may become necessary. The tendons can be lengthened or an arthroplasty, an operation in which a small portion of bone is removed in order to straighten the toe, can be performed.

FALLEN ARCHES

If your feet hurt during the day or quickly grow tired when you're standing, then your longitudinal arches are probably weakening.

Constant standing, uncomfortable shoes and obesity all contribute to the breakdown of the ligaments that hold the foot together. When your arches give way, the imbalance causes tension in your lower back. Lower back pain is, in fact, a common sign of fallen arches.

One way to relieve and prevent fallen arches is to exercise your feet. Toe curling, stretching, and foot rotation will help. An orthotic device may provide extra support.

NEUROMAS

Although we've discussed neuromas in connection with other problems, this condition is common enough in the aging foot to merit its own section.

The word *neuroma* (*neur* means *nerve*; *oma* means *tumor*) is actually a misnomer. Neuromas aren't cancer-like tumors caused by abnormally developing cells. They're thickened nerve tissue caused by chronic pressure on the nerve, and they occur most often in the weight-bearing ball of the foot near the toe joint.

A neuroma can be caused by high-heeled shoes, by a thinning fat pad or by a biomechanical disorder.

Feet naturally spread when you walk so even normally-fitting shoes are somewhat constricting. If your shoes are too narrow or your feet are especially sensitive, the constant squeeze will irritate the bursas (fluid-filled sacs cushioning the joints), tendons, blood vessels and nerves in the ball of the foot. The bursas and nerves swell and eventually thicken and become permanently scarred.

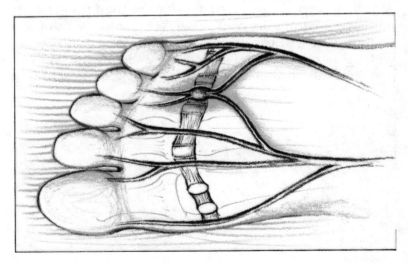

Neuromas are caused by pressure on a nerve. Soaking alternately in warm and cool water and wearing wider shoes are often helpful.

The space between the weight-bearing bones in your foot is very small and the thickened nerve fills the space and is then pressed by the bones. The resulting pain usually occurs around the third and fourth toes and is often described as a stabbing, burning, pins-and-needles pain that shoots out toward the toes and sometimes up the back of the leg.

Sometimes neuromas cause painful foot cramps, usually after you wear shoes for a few hours. These are not the usual cramps; the toes do not change position as in a muscle cramp. Even if you massage your foot until it relaxes, it will cramp again as soon as you put your shoe on because the cramp is caused by your shoe irritating the afflicted nerve in the muscle of your foot.

You can treat a neuroma at home with contrasting soaks. Soak your foot alternately for five minutes in warm and two minutes in cool water for about 20 minutes, ending with a warm water soak. You might also wear wider shoes (though not so wide they slip off your heel as you walk) and use in-shoe padding to relieve pressure.

HEEL PROBLEMS

7

Time wounds all heels.
—*Jane Ace*, Goodman Ace;
The Fine Art of Hypochondria;
Or, How Are You?

HEEL SPURS

Heel spurs are the best known heel problems. A heel spur is a point of excess bone growth on the heel. The calcium extends either toward the toes, from the bottom of the heel, or back toward the Achilles tendon. Heel spurs can be confirmed only by X ray.

Warm soaks and rest will soothe painful heel spurs. A prescribed orthotic device can provide support. If the spur is particularly painful, your doctor might also inject the area with a steroid for immediate relief.

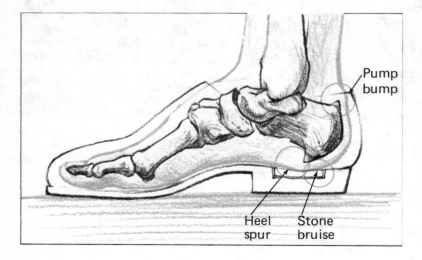

Pump bumps, stone bruises and spurs are common heel problems. Avoiding shoes that irritate can help. For severe pain, consult with your doctor.

If the pain is severe, you might need to have the spur removed. Accurate and correct surgical procedure can minimize damage to the bone and ligament but it still takes at least six weeks to recover from heel surgery.

PLANTAR FASCIITIS

The most common heel problem is the painful tearing of plantar fascia connecting the toes and heel. (*Plantar* means bottom of the foot and *fascia* means dense fibrous tissue.)

If your foot flattens or becomes unstable over time, or if your shoes wear in a way that stretches this long ligament, it will begin to pull away from its attachment to the heel and cause swelling and pain. The pain is especially noticeable when you push off with your toes while walking since this movement stretches the already inflamed ligament. Without treatment, the fibers of the ligament attached to the heel will become more swollen and cause pain around the heel. The pain is usually centered slightly in front of the heel toward the arch.

This condition is terribly disabling because, to avoid pain, you'll probably try to walk on your toes—the best way to further tear the fascia and to increase your pain. In fact, victims of plantar fasciitis occasionally injure the ligament in the healthy foot while walking on their toes to avoid pain in the afflicted foot.

The first step in treating plantar fasciitis is to reduce the swelling and pain. Alternating warm and cold water soaks, using an anti-inflammatory drug like aspirin and cushioning the foot with a soft insole will help reduce the strain and swelling. But total rest is necessary to heal a torn ligament, so the best treatment is to not use your foot at all.

A doctor may use local anesthetics to relieve the pain and prescribe anti-inflammatory medication to relieve swelling. He or she might also recommend strappings and paddings to stabilize the foot to reduce stress on the ligament. Sometimes a walker, cane or light cast is used to rest the foot completely.

Once swelling and pain are under control, you can massage the bottom of your foot with a foot roller or an empty soda bottle, gently rolling it back and forth along the bottom of the foot to relax the ligament and muscles. Deep massage with the fingers will also help relieve muscle spasms.

Plantar fasciitis is rarely treated surgically. An orthotic device (in-shoe support) can be prescribed to stabilize your foot and prevent a recurrence. Over 90 percent of the time heel spurs and plantar fasciitis can be controlled with an in-shoe orthotic device which cups the heel. This prevents the plantar fascia from spreading. It also supports the arch to prevent lengthening of the plantar fascia and allows the inflammation to calm down. For most heel problems, a well-supported shoe with a firm shank and a moderate heel lift is better than a soft flat shoe.

PUMP BUMPS

Pump bumps, caused by abnormal heel motion, are an especially irritating form of heel spur because they occur at the point where the Achilles tendon connects with your heel and are rubbed by the heel counter in your shoe. This rubbing can cause painful heel bursitis and even tendonitis of the Achilles tendon.

Treatment consists mainly of protecting the heel from further rubbing against the shoe by wearing a larger shoe equipped with a heel lift to stabilize the foot.

The best solution to pump bumps is to wear shoes that don't irritate the heel, but if the pump bump continues to be a source of pain, you'll probably need professional treatment.

Your doctor can supply therapeutic injections or anti-inflammatory medications to relieve pain temporarily, and physical therapies like ultrasound and other heat treatments will also relieve pain. Pump bumps can be removed surgically, but again, heel surgery can require up to six weeks for recovery and is accompanied by a certain amount of pain. Surgery should be considered only a last resort.

"STONE BRUISE"

A "stone bruise" is a bruised heel bone. It's usually caused by direct trauma to the heel such as stepping or jumping on something sharp.

The pain of a stone bruise is usually felt in the center of the heel and is aggravated by pressure on the injured bone.

Like a fracture, a stone bruise is an injury to the bone. Unlike a fracture, it will probably heal itself if it's allowed to rest.

Treat the bruise with ice packs for the first two or three days. Keep the foot elevated as much as possible and stay off it. It might even be helpful to use crutches or a walker for a few days. Additional cushioning of the heel bone should help.

8

THE RIGHT SHOE
FOR THE RIGHT FOOT
(AND FOR THE LEFT)

To a foot in a shoe the whole world seems to be paved with leather.
—The Hitopadesa, I, *c. 500*

Anthropologists have discovered high-heeled shoes in the tombs of the pharaohs. Even in those distant days, shoes served not only to protect the feet, but to adorn them. High style was the dubious privilege of the upper classes, however. Paintings in Egyptian tombs show royal women wearing high-heeled shoes while servants milled about in flat, utilitarian sandals.

Most shoes are still designed with fashion rather than function in mind. We spend $60 to $70 billion a year on shoes in the U.S. The average woman owns ten pairs of shoes, the average man owns six and the average American child goes through two or three new pairs a year.

From spiked heels to running shoes, style comes first in footwear design. The most artfully and expensively made shoe can irritate your foot if it hurts you when you walk.

Most shoes purchased are machine-made, but you can also buy orthopedic shoes (ready-made shoes adaptable to some extent to your foot) or custom-fitted, molded shoes if your feet have special needs.

SHOPPING FOR SHOES

Looking for new shoes can be discouraging. Some shoe store personnel aren't trained to properly fit your feet, and many will tell you an uncomfortable shoe just needs breaking in. To add to your confusion, shoes that feel great on the store's soft carpet may hurt later when you wear them on concrete or linoleum. Besides, most of us are looking for shoes that are both attractive and comfortable—a tall order, especially if you're a woman. How many women have *you* seen dressed-for-success in the pages of fashion magazines sporting a brand new pair of comfortable oxfords?

The most important and most elusive quality in a pair of shoes is proper fit. Why is good fit elusive? Because shoes come in a few standard sizes and feet come in an infinite number of not-so-standard sizes. There is no average foot and no two feet are shaped alike. Even your feet differ from one another in size and shape, and they are constantly changing.

Another obstacle to good fit is that different styles are shaped differently and therefore tend to fit differently. Because you wear a size nine in one style is no guarantee that you can wear a size nine in another.

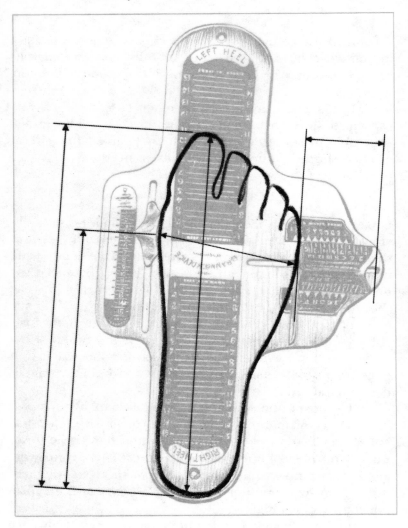

Whenever you buy new shoes, have your feet measured. This device measures both length and width.

And what does size nine mean anyway? Believe it or not, shoe size is still based on a 14th-century king's decree that three barleycorns would equal an inch and that 39 barleycorns (or 13 inches) would be the largest normal foot size. Men's size 13 is still the largest size most shoe stores carry and it is still 13 inches long. Other sizes still vary by a third of an inch (one barleycorn) so that size 12 is 12⅔ inches long, size 11 is 12⅓ inches long, etc.

Complicating life further, some manufacturers write shoe sizes in code. The size known to the layperson as 7½A is written 175, for instance. The first number of the code indicates width:

$$0 = AA$$
$$1 = A$$
$$2 = B$$
$$3 = C$$
$$4 = D$$
$$5 = E$$
$$6 = EE$$

and the remaining numbers indicate length. If the last number is 0, the shoe size is a full size. If the last number is 5, the shoe is a half-size. Thus 3120 is a 12C and 165 is a 6½A.

Shoe sizing is necessarily somewhat arbitrary. No shoemaker could afford to make shoes in every possible shape and size, and shoe stores can't afford to stock each of the styles they carry in all sizes. In fact, the more expensive the style, the fewer sizes your dealer can afford to have on hand.

But you can find shoes to fit your feet if you're willing to spend some time shopping for them. Choose a shoe-store that is reputable and will give you a cash refund, if necessary, for unmarred shoes.

Always insist that both your feet be measured for both length and width. Have them measured while you're standing because feet tend to spread when they're carrying your full weight. If your feet tend to swell, shop for shoes late in the day. One of your feet is probably longer than the other; always fit your larger foot. You can fill in the other shoe with an inner sole, if necessary.

How do you know when shoes fit? First, don't listen to any salesperson who tells you a stiff, uncomfortable pair of shoes needs to be broken in. Always try both shoes on. If they fit, they'll feel right. If they're uncomfortable, they don't fit.

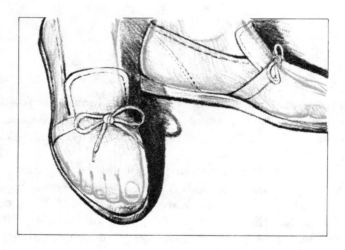

Choose shoes that fit well. The fit should be snug but not too tight across the widest part of the foot. There should be a little space in front of the toes, and the heel should fit well without slipping.

Walk around in the shoes. Be sure there is no excess pressure on the toes or the ball of the foot. Your heel should fit snugly, but the back of the shoe (the counter) shouldn't rub against your Achilles tendon. The top of the toe box should be high enough to allow your toes to move. The shoe should be flexible enough to bend easily at the proper place, but it shouldn't dig into your foot above your big toe joint.

Proper fit starts at the ball of your foot, the widest part. The shoe should fit snugly across the ball of your foot without being constricting. Stand in the shoes and have the salesperson try to pinch the top of the shoe. The leather should be able to be rippled slightly for about 1/4 inch above the top of the foot.

Take off the shoes and run your hand along the insides to make sure there are no wrinkles, ridges, loose linings or other irregularities that might eventually irritate your foot.

Take the shoes home and wear them around the house for two hours. Cover them with a pair of old socks to protect the soles. Spend the time doing something active so you'll know just how comfortable the shoes are under any conditions. If they're uncomfortable, return them and start looking again.

A pair of shoes is a substantial investment, especially if you're on a fixed income. It's worth a bit of trouble to evaluate them thoroughly for fit and comfort.

THE PERFECT SHOE

The shoe the experts most often recommend is a light-weight, flexible, leather shoe with a lace. Avoid reptile skins, patent leathers and plastics. They don't breathe, and your feet tend to overheat and form sweaty breeding grounds inside them for fungi and bacteria.

Leather and fabric uppers are good because they breathe and tend to be cooler. Leather is still the most durable and the coolest material for soles if you live in the country. But it doesn't absorb the shock of walking on pavement as well as rubber and crepe soles do. If you do wear shoes with rubber or crepe soles, be sure the uppers are either fabric or are perforated because these materials can be uncomfortably warm. Canvas sneakers are ideal for this reason.

Leather is the most durable lining but cotton is good if your feet sweat a lot. The lining in the heel, called the heel counter, should be leather or plastic. Some shoes come with cardboard heel counters which quickly deteriorate.

The ideal shoe raises your heel no more than an inch and a half above the ball of your foot. It has a heel that's square or rectangular and that extends at least a quarter inch beyond the sides of the shoe to give it plenty of contact with the ground, stabilizing your foot as you walk. Rubber heels give much better shock absorption and do not slip as easily as leather.

High-heeled shoes force your pelvis forward and your shoulders back causing swayback, straining the muscles in your legs and thighs, and often causing backaches. They also force the back of the foot up, often shortening the Achilles tendon, and force the toes to reach lower, stretching the tendons in the front of the foot and often causing crippling pain in later years. Because they shift your weight to the front of your foot, they usually cause a thick, sometimes painful callus to form on the ball of the foot.

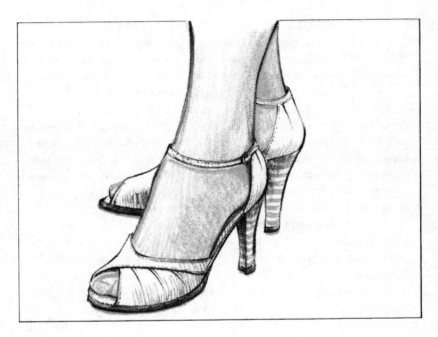

Shoes with heels over two inches high put excess pressure on the front of your foot. They can cause calluses and bursitis as well as back problems.

The extra weight also puts pressure on the joints between the toe bones and can cause bursitis, a swelling of the water-filled bursal sacs overlaying the joints, or hallux valgus, a turning in of the big toe joint that is often the precursor of bunions.

If you must wear a heel, wear one no more than two inches high. You may need to change your heel height frequently during the day, but never change more than $\frac{1}{2}''$ at a time. If you have back pains with one heel height, consider another.

High heels are not the only problem with women's shoes. Nobody's feet are pointed in the center, but many women's dress shoes come with pointed toes that force your toes into a tight little bunch causing bunions, corns, calluses, and bursitis. Even women's square-toed shoes are often too flat in the toe box, and the top of the shoe presses down on the toes. Often, too, the soles in women's shoes are narrower than the sole of the foot and cause permanent fissures and creases on the bottom of the foot as well as soft corns between the toes. Constant constriction of the sole can also result in neuromas.

Many podiatrists recommend low-heeled, open-toed sandals. The toes are unconstricted, and you don't have to worry about fitting the heel because the strap can be adjusted.

Boots are usually too hot to wear all day. When you buy them, be sure they're not too tight around your calves or around your ankles and that they aren't too heavy. Make sure the heels are not too high.

The shank of the shoe runs from the heel to the ball and consists of a sturdy outer sole, an inside layer of material that gives the shank its shape and an inner sole to cushion the foot. It's the sloping part of the shoe that conforms to the bottom of the foot under the arch.

The higher the heel, the greater the slope of the shank. A shank from the heel to the ball of the foot should be firm and difficult to bend. Cheap materials like pressed cardboard don't provide enough support and usually break down, bending in the middle of the shoe where the foot isn't meant to bend. An inadequate shank probably causes more foot problems than any other part of the shoe.

SOCKS AND STOCKINGS

Ill-fitting shoes aren't the only instruments you can use to torture your feet. Tight elastic stockings can pull on the toes and contract the foot, aggravating chronic conditions like hammertoes. Nylon irritates the skin, causes a lot of friction and doesn't absorb moisture well. If you do wear nylon stockings, wear a cotton half-sock under them. And don't wear elastic one-size-fits-all stockings; it's better to buy stockings in specific sizes. Avoid garters or garter belts that constrict the calf or thigh, especially if you have circulatory problems in your feet or legs. Cotton socks are the best, of course, and if you can't find 100 percent cotton, try to find a cotton blend. Wool socks are great for cold weather and you can wear them to bed at night if your feet get cold. Be sure you buy your socks long enough and that they're preshrunk. Tight socks can be as irritating to your feet as tight shoes.

ORTHOPEDIC SHOES

Orthopedic shoes sold in special stores can be fitted to feet with minor problems. Usually these shoes are extra-wide, extra-deep or made of extremely soft material. They can also be a combination last, with a narrow heel and a wide ball of the foot, for instance.

Orthopedic shoes look like standard shoes but are specially adapted to specific foot variations. They can provide extra room for conditions like bunions or severe hammertoes.

Usually these shoes are supplemented with a soft innersole for extra protection. They're usually prescribed by a podiatrist and are more expensive than standard shoes.

CUSTOM-FITTED, MOLDED SHOES

When foot problems are severely debilitating or deforming, or when severe diabetes, circulatory problems or arthritis make your foot sensitive to the slightest pressure, custom-fitted shoes are a must.

Molded shoes used to be very heavy but the new ones are light, durable, soft and often more attractive than the old versions.

Molded shoes always require a cast molding by a shoe specialist such as a podiatrist or pedorthotist (shoe maker). Plaster is poured into a negative cast and the result is a replica of your foot, called a positive cast. The shoes are molded to this plaster model of your foot and adapted to accommodate any problems you might have. They can be useful if your feet differ markedly from one another in size or shape. Diabetics can use them if standard shoes are causing chronic ulcerations. Arthritics whose feet are held in permanent contraction and whose fat pads are practically nonexistent often find them comfortable.

Custom-fitted shoes can help you walk if you can't undergo corrective foot surgery and suffer from chronic conditions like ulcers, infections and painful corns and calluses.

The main drawback of these shoes is that they're very expensive, though after the first pair has been made, the plaster cast can be re-used and subsequent pairs will be cheaper. The same cast can generally be used for several years as long as the structure of your foot does not change.

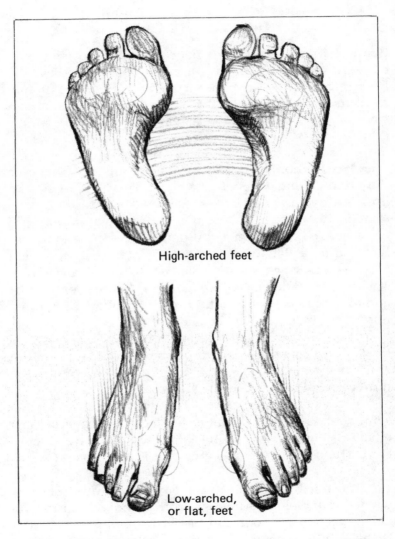

High-arched feet

Low-arched, or flat, feet

People with high arches often develop hammertoes, corns and plantar calluses. Flat feet often develop bunions and arch pain.

ORTHOTIC DEVICES

Biomechanics is a relatively new branch of medicine concerned with the dynamics of human motion. Studies have been done on the range of normal and abnormal motion to control the foot's range of motion and eliminate pain caused by imbalances and excessive motion with orthotic devices.

Orthoses are shoe inserts molded to your foot. They're commonly confused with arch supports sold over the counter and through the mail. They're designed to improve the function of the feet and legs based on the relationship of each part of the foot to the ground.

They're made from a cast mold of the foot and manufactured as a flat form to fit into a standard shoe, and they're prescribed by a podiatrist. The podiatrist prescribes certain degrees of wedging for the front of the foot and for the rear of the foot. This helps your foot to function better by improving its stability.

The first type is called a rigid functional orthosis. It is made of high-tensile-strength plastic for athletes, children and other people with excessively flexible feet to limit the movement of the foot in the shoe.

The second type (and the type most practical for the aging foot) is a molded leather and cork device. It is most effective, however, if the heels are less than two inches high. The cork and leather material is an excellent shock absorber.

The third type of orthosis is the accommodative or padded innersole. It's made of soft rubber or plastic and helps cushion the foot that has lost much of its fat pad. Diabetes and arthritis sufferers can often use this form of support. Padded innersoles don't control or balance the foot; they simply relieve friction and are the most popular orthoses.

Don't let a shoe salesperson try to improve the fit of a shoe that is too large by selling you metatarsal pads or cookies (concave shells inserted under your arch) or a scaphoid raise (a convex piece of rubber also inserted under your arch). All these fillers do is decrease the space available to your feet. They do nothing about repositioning your feet properly, and they can damage your feet. Altering the position of one part of your foot can throw the rest of your foot, leg, or back out of balance.

Over-the-counter arch supports have some limited practical value. Sometimes people with tired feet feel better with extra cushioning in their shoes, but that is the extent of the usefulness of the simple arch support. Normal feet don't need arch supports because the arch doesn't bear any weight. If you've ever seen your footprint in the sand, you've probably noticed that your arch doesn't leave much of an impression. A mass-produced arch support is of no use in correcting the specific problems of abnormal feet.

9

THE ARTHRITIC FOOT

I am interested in physical medicine
because my father was. I am interested
in medical research because I believe in it.
I am interested in arthritis because I have it.
—Bernard M. Baruch

The word *arthritis* is used to describe a number of joint abnormalities. An increase or decrease in the space between the bones, a breakdown of part of the bone or the growth of small, needle-shaped particles called osteophytes around the joint can all be the results of an arthritic condition.

There are at least 100 forms of arthritis but the most common are osteoarthritis, rheumatoid arthritis and gout. These forms of arthritis don't affect only the feet. However, they are more common in the feet because of the large network of bones subject to so much wear and tear.

OSTEOARTHRITIS

The most common form of arthritis, osteoarthritis, affects about half of all arthritis sufferers. Also called degenerative joint disease or wear-and-tear arthritis, it is associated with aging.

As we grow older, the cartilage around our joints deteriorates slowly. It initially develops thin cracks that later become deep fissures and is eventually eroded. Without this protective cartilage, bones rub against one another, irritating the nerves and often causing aching or more intense pain in the joints. This rubbing can also stimulate the development of bone spurs that often enlarge the joint and make it painful and stiff.

Osteoarthritis usually develops gradually and affects the tips of the fingers and the weight-bearing joints, the joint under the big toe for instance. Traumatic osteoarthritis seems to develop in joints that have been injured— the ankle is a favorite site—years after the actual injury occurred.

No one seems to know why some people develop osteoarthritis more acutely than others or why women are affected slightly more often than men. Two people whose X rays show the same degree of joint deterioration often experience markedly different symptoms. One might experience intense pain while the other experiences no symptoms at all.

Osteoarthritis is rarely crippling and although the joints are often enlarged, stiff and painful with this disease, they are rarely inflamed as in other, more serious forms of arthritis.

ARTHRITIS DO'S AND DON'TS

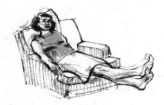

Take a break from physical activity every ten or twenty minutes.

Don't slouch or sit in one position for too long. Walk around frequently.

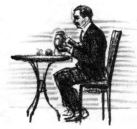

Do recommended exercises daily. Don't let regular activities replace exercises.

Sit while working to lessen stress on joints.

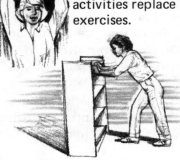

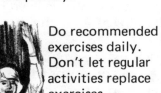

Choose comfort. For instance, use a shoulder bag to avoid stress on fingers.

Instead of pulling large objects, push with your palms to avoid stress on fingers.

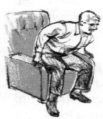

Do ease in and out of a chair gently.

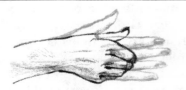

Exercise daily.

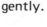

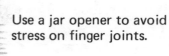

Use a jar opener to avoid stress on finger joints.

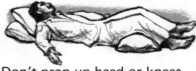

Don't prop up head or knees at night. This may ease the pain for the moment, but you will be stiff and sore when you awake.

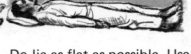

Do lie as flat as possible. Use a small pillow or no pillow at all.

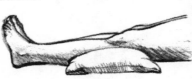

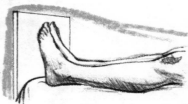

If knees are swollen, sandbags will prevent feet from turning out and putting stress on knees.

If ankles or toes are swollen, use a board or frame to prop up blankets and sheets.

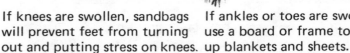

Because there is little soft tissue swelling with osteoarthritis, anti-inflammatory drugs provide short-term relief.
Surgery is often used to treat advanced cases; spurs and
other bony particles can be removed or the joint can be
replaced with an artificial implant.

If the afflicted joint isn't too painful, exercise is important in preventing muscle deterioration. Strengthening the
muscles around the joint can provide a certain amount of
support and relieve some of the pressure on the joint. Try
the exercises in Chapter 13 and do as much walking as you
can. You can also massage your feet with foot rollers or
with an empty soft drink bottle, gently rolling it back and
forth with each foot two or three times a day.

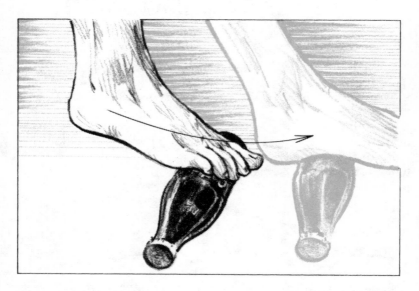

Gently rolling a bottle with your foot will stimulate circulation.

Foot soaks can also relieve arthritic pain and stiffness. When your feet are stiff but not swollen, soak them in warm water for 15 minutes once or twice a day. When they are swollen *and* stiff, soak them for five minutes in warm water followed by two minutes in cool water. Soak for another five minutes in warm water and end with the two-minute cool-water soak. This can relieve discomfort very effectively if you do it twice a day.

Be wary of therapies advertised as miracle cures in the back pages of magazines and newspapers. All arthritic medicine should be prescribed by your doctor. Your doctor might also administer ultrasound or heat treatment. (See Chapter 17, "Physical Therapy.")

RHEUMATOID ARTHRITIS

Rheumatoid arthritis affects about one in five arthritis victims and afflicts women three times more often than men.

It is characterized by inflammation; the joints are painful, stiff, swollen, tender and often warm to the touch. Stiffness and pain might be most intense in the morning after a night of lying motionless in bed. Stiffness can recur throughout the day either as the result of intense use of the joint or as the result of not using it at all.

Rheumatoid arthritis is also often accompanied by the feeling of being generally ill, including loss of appetite, weight loss, weakness, exhaustion and a low-grade fever.

Though it's often mild, rheumatoid arthritis can be disabling. The inflammation begins with no apparent cause in the joint lining and eventually begins to destroy nearby cartilage and underlying bone. Without treatment, surrounding muscles and other soft tissues are sometimes damaged and can pull the bones out of alignment with one another to deform the joint. Scar tissue sometimes forms between bone ends and can fuse the joint, making it permanently immovable. Inflammation can also cause joint distortion with toes veering off at unnatural angles. Severe joint distortion is usually painful but there are people with badly deformed joints who experience very little pain and are able to function normally.

Though rheumatoid arthritis is a serious illness, experts agree that, with appropriate treatment in the first year, most people improve substantially and have fewer symptoms. This condition can become disabling, however, even with proper medical care.

Many rheumatologists say that even severe cases of rheumatoid arthritis can be successfully treated if the victim continues to walk. Obviously, keeping the feet functional means a great deal in controlling this disease.

No one knows what causes rheumatoid arthritis but there is new evidence that genes might have something to do with it. Acute recurrences seem to occur during periods of stress, but there's no convincing evidence that stress causes rheumatoid arthritis. Proper alignment of the foot to correct the imbalance which occurs in rheumatoid arthritis requires primary foot care and general medical care together.

Aspirin is often recommended to relieve the pain and swelling of rheumatoid arthritis in doses of twelve to twenty-five tablets a day. Sometimes anti-inflammatory steroids like cortisone are injected into the painful areas to reduce swelling and pain.

GOUT

Gout is the painful result of crystals of uric acid—a chemical made by the liver and passed out of the body in the urine—settling in and around joint tissues. The big toe joint, a favorite site for arthritis, is eventually affected in most cases of gout probably because it is subject to so much pressure in walking.

Gout is a chronic disease and usually consists of recurring attacks followed by periods of remission. Though some people never have more than one attack, most victims suffer repeated attacks throughout their lives. An attack can come on rapidly within an hour or two and can last from eight to ten days. The joint becomes very painful, swollen, hot and tender. The skin above it reddens and sometimes even turns purple.

Gout is thought to be hereditary. It occurs when the body is unable to dissolve uric acid crystals in the blood and deposits them in the joints.

Uric acid buildup can be the result of faulty kidney function because the kidney normally filters out extra uric acid. It can also be the result of abnormal purine metabolism. Purines are the protein compounds that form uric acid crystals and they're found in foods like anchovies, sardines and other shellfish and organ meats.

The use of diuretics ("water pills"), a rapid loss of tissues from crash dieting, or the destruction of a tumor can also cause uric acid to accumulate in the bloodstream. This condition is called "pseudo-gout."

Uric acid crystals settle out of the bloodstream in every part of the body but the brain and the nerves. The damage is caused by crystal deposits in the kidneys, in the blood vessels, around the tendons and in the joints.

There is no cure for gout, but it can be controlled. Colchicine, a drug made from parts of the autumn crocus, has been used since ancient Egyptian days to relieve the pain of gout and to prevent its recurrence.

Your doctor might treat your condition with an anti-inflammatory drug, with probenecid which increases uric acid excretion or with allopurinol which reduces uric acid production. Steroid injections can relieve pain but don't treat the cause. On the other hand, a nerve block injection at the ankle can reduce extreme foot pain.

Rest during a gout attack and keep your body weight off the affected joints. Drink plenty of water, up to three quarts a day, to dilute the uric acid salts in the kidneys. Soak the painful joint in cool water every hour or two for five minutes at a time.

When your joint is so badly damaged that it no longer functions, surgery to remodel the joint or to replace it with an artificial implant can restore most of your lost mobility.

COLD FEET

10

A man is as old as his arteries.
—*Thomas Sydenham*

It makes sense that we use the expression "cold feet" to describe fear. Tension is one of the many conditions that can constrict the tiny capillaries that nourish the skin and nerves of our extremities, and poor circulation causes cold feet.

Why do cold feet occur more often with age? Because we become more vulnerable to the conditions that disrupt circulation: hardening of the arteries, varicose veins, diabetes, heart disease and lymphatic problems. And because we're finally paying for the thousands of cigarettes smoked and cups of coffee consumed. Like fear, caffeine and nicotine constrict the skin's tiny irrigation system.

WHY FEET SUFFER FIRST

Arteries are the vessels that carry fresh, nutrient-rich blood from the heart to the rest of the body.

The central arterial system feeds the heart, brain, kidneys, liver and other vital organs. The peripheral artery system feeds everything else. It's peripheral because impairing the circulation to these body parts is not immediately life-threatening.

The peripheral artery system is also divided into two systems. The superficial artery system nourishes the skin and the area just beneath the skin. The deep artery system feeds the muscles, nerves, tendons, bones and joints.

When any circulatory problem develops, the body shuts off the superficial system in order to divert blood to the more critical deep artery system. That's why skin, hair and nail changes are the first signs of poor circulation. Because the feet are so far from the heart, they're affected by reduced circulation first. And because circulation is what maintains our body temperature, reduced circulation means cold feet.

Undernourished feet are not necessarily serious themselves, but it's important to pay attention to them because they can be the first signs of serious disorders.

CARING FOR COLD FEET

Undernourished feet are usually more sensitive to irritation. Ulcers, corns and calluses are more common in feet with poor circulation, for instance.

Exercise is the best way to stimulate circulation. When you walk or run, the muscles in your foot massage it from the inside.

Avoid coffee and cigarettes. They restrict circulation. In cold weather, wool socks can keep your feet warm and soaking your feet in warm water for 15 minutes can warm them up if they've developed a chill.

Your doctor can prescribe drugs that temporarily open up the small blood vessels to stimulate circulation and relieve the chilly feeling. You should see a doctor in any case if you have a general circulation problem.

HARDENING OF THE ARTERIES

Arteriosclerosis is a disease in which the arteries are narrowed or blocked by deposits of fatty tissues on their inner walls. It especially threatens the flow of blood to the feet when it affects the major artery that branches just below the abdomen into the tributaries that feed the legs.

When this artery begins to narrow, one or both of your legs and feet will ache and cramp when you walk. This cramping is called intermittent claudication— intermittent because it occurs only with activity and goes away when you rest your foot and leg. The narrowed artery causes cramping because not enough blood is flowing through it to supply the leg and foot muscles with the oxygen they need to function. As the disease progresses, you're able to walk shorter and shorter distances before cramping occurs. Intermittent claudication is a major symptom of arteriosclerosis.

As arteriosclerosis progresses, your foot and leg will probably begin to ache and cramp while you're resting and even while you're asleep. This nocturnal cramping is called night recumbency leg cramping and can be so painful you might need to get up and walk around to relieve the spasms.

Poor circulation in your feet means that the skin is deprived of oxygen. As a result it grows thin and loses its hair. Toenails often become brittle and develop chips and ridges. Calluses thicken, and small, painful ulcers develop on the toes, the heel or the top of the foot.

Although severe arteriosclerosis requires a doctor's care, you can help reduce night recumbency cramping at home by exercising before you go to bed and when you get up in the morning. Take a walk and try the exercise routines in Chapter 13. Vitamins, especially C and E are often helpful. You can take Vitamin E, in natural form, at bedtime to relieve cramping.

Your doctor might send you to a vascular specialist who will evaluate the degree to which your artery is blocked. Treatment depends on the severity of the blockage and can be a blood-thinning medicine, physical therapy to stimulate circulation or surgery to remove the fatty deposits or to replace the afflicted section of the artery.

Even if you don't have arteriosclerosis, avoid wearing anything that constricts your legs or feet. Don't wear clothes that pinch or bind. Avoid girdles, belts, garters, boots and elastic stockings, including support hose, unless prescribed. Give up smoking and lose weight if you have a weight problem. Not only does excess weight strain already overworked blood vessels, it creates layers of fat that use up an already limited supply of oxygen. Don't sit in uncomfortable or cramped positions; don't cross your legs, for example. Avoid extreme temperatures. Heat increases the body's demand for oxygen, and cold constricts the blood vessels.

Twice a day, relax your feet in a tub of warm water.

Never use hot water because it increases the need of the feet for oxygen. Massage your feet underwater and clean them with a mild soap. After the bath, apply rubbing alcohol to your feet followed by a coat of a lanolin-based cream and some talc.

Do adopt a low-fat diet. Your doctor will probably prescribe such a diet for you to slow the further blockage of your arteries.

Walk whenever possible and massage your feet to stimulate circulation.

VARICOSE VEINS

Veins are the vessels that return the blood from your feet to your heart. There are valves spaced regularly along the veins that constantly open and close to help the blood defy gravity on its return trip and to prevent backflow.

When one of these valves weakens, it allows blood to flow back down and collect at the lower valve, weakening all the valves in the area in a kind of domino effect. The veins swell and show up as blue or brown discolorations under the skin.

Varicose veins are often hereditary, but they can also be caused by obesity and the pressure excess weight exerts on the veins in the legs. Due to pregnancy and childbearing, women have varicose veins more often than men. When the condition consists only of enlarged veins, it doesn't usually pose serious problems. But when the valves in the veins begin to break down, blood collects below the valves faster than it can be pumped away. The blood pools in the foot and leg and stagnates. The foot responds by slowly swelling, especially when you're sitting or standing for prolonged periods. The skin of your foot thickens and loses hair and is more sensitive to irritation. Often the skin feels itchy because of the pooling of blood and stretching of the skin. The skin is so fragile that scratching it can cause serious ulcerations. Poor circulation makes the skin an ideal breeding ground for infection.

Wearing elastic support hose and elevating your feet above heart level will encourage blood to return to the heart. Walking and the simple exercises described in Chapter 13 will also stimulate circulation.

If your varicose veins are severe, your doctor might strip the veins. The effect is to divert the blood that has

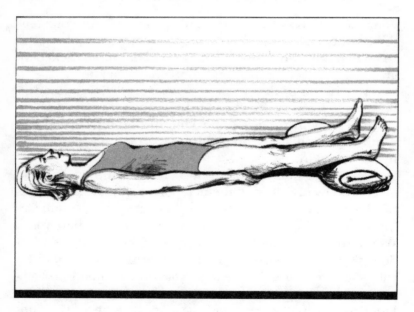

Elevating your feet above heart level will improve blood flow.

been stagnating in the damaged superficial veins to the stronger, deeper veins in your leg in order to improve circulation.

LYMPH INFECTIONS

The lymph system is a system of glands that secrete lymph—a fluid that circulates through the body tissues and fights infections. When an infection in your foot progresses to infect your lymph system, the result is a serious condition called lymphangitis that requires immediate medical attention. Its symptoms are greatly swollen feet and reddish streaks along your legs.

In other conditions where there is no infection, the longer the swelling is left untreated, the greater the chance that lymphatic tissue will harden and cause permanent damage. This is known as lymphedema.

To treat this condition, your doctor will probably compress your foot with bandages to prevent swelling. Physical therapy and massage are also useful and sometimes even electric currents are used to cause muscle contractions and circulate the lymph.

11

FRACTURES AND SPRAINS

Healing is a matter of time,
but sometimes also a matter of opportunity.
—Hippocrates, 460 – 400 B.C.

Why do fractures, strains and sprains seem to take longer to heal when we're older? Why, as we age, do we also grow more afraid of falling, of breaking hips, ankles and feet?

There is a myth that old bones never heal; the stories are of aging aunts, cousins and grandparents who fell down the stairs, broke their hips and never really recovered. To this day, the fables go, the victims hobble painfully on a cane, if at all.

The simple truth is that healing often does take longer, especially when calcium is depleted and circulation slows down. Slow healing, though, does not mean incomplete healing. Most body tissues replenish themselves constantly.

OSTEOPOROSIS (MINERAL DEPLETION OF BONES)

Bone tissue is made mostly of a soft protein framework and calcium salt deposits on the frame. Your body routinely loses calcium and replaces it by absorbing it from food.

But when bones are depleted of calcium as they are in the condition called osteoporosis, they become brittle, break more easily and heal more slowly. There are a number of factors that can cause osteoporosis in aging bones.

The female hormone estrogen and the male hormone androgen help maintain calcium balance. Their production declines at mid-life.

As we grow older, life-long dietary deficiencies catch up with us. Most of us have probably never eaten enough calcium-rich foods.

Osteoporosis is not an inevitable accompaniment to aging, however.

Exercise is the most effective way to prevent calcium depletion. Stress makes bones grow thicker and tougher. Osteoporosis can also be treated with estrogen, but the use of any medication should be discussed with your doctor.

While you're working on rebuilding brittle, weakened bones, soft-soled shoes with orthotic devices prescribed by your podiatrist can cushion your feet and prevent stress fractures.

TREATMENT FOR FRACTURES

It's important to have any broken foot bone set immediately. The pieces of an untreated fracture might not grow together, with painful and disabling results. This non-union can require surgery to fuse the bone. Sometimes metal plates, pins, or screws are used to reunite the separate pieces.

Depending on the size of the broken bone and whether or not it's a weight-bearing bone, a fracture can take six to twelve weeks to heal.

You should not have to wear a cast that long, however. Once the bone has set in the first few weeks, the bone can be held in proper alignment with a combination of strapping and a semi-rigid support molded for the fracture site.

But there is more to healing a fracture than resting the bone. When you don't use a muscle for even a week, it begins to deteriorate. While it's in the cast, the muscle can be stimulated with ultrasound and other physical therapy techniques to help maintain muscle tone.

When the cast or wrapping is removed, however, it's time for you to do some active healing. You need to exercise your foot using some of the exercises suggested in Chapter 13. Walking is also a great way to strengthen injured feet.

Strengthening your foot is important not only to heal it completely, but also to prevent new fractures. When a bone has not been used for a few weeks, it loses strength and is more susceptible to stress fractures.

While healing you can stay in shape with other exercises like swimming that don't put weight on your feet.

STRAINS AND SPRAINS

Tendons are elastic structures that connect muscles to bone. A strain is a damaged muscle, tendon, or tendon sheath.

Ligaments connect bones at joints and keep your joints from moving too freely. It's normal for your foot to move inward or outward, but when you exceed the normal joint range of motion, you can tear the ligaments on the inside or outside of your ankle. A torn or twisted ligament is called a sprain.

Sprains are the most common ankle injuries. You can sprain your ankle falling down steps or just twisting your foot on an uneven section of sidewalk.

The most common ankle sprain is an inversion sprain in which the foot turns in and under the leg. The injury is just below the ankle joint on the outside of the foot. Often your whole foot and ankle swell and turn black-and-blue.

Eversion sprains, in which the foot turns out, are much less common. They frequently result in a fracture of the ankle bone.

Sprained ankles and feet are among the most neglected injuries. Even a mild sprain can cause more trouble than a fracture if it isn't treated immediately. An untreated sprain can cause life-long ankle instability.

If you twist your ankle and can't walk off the pain in five minutes, assume it's sprained. Elevate your foot as soon as you can and wrap it in a mildly compressed elastic bandage. Call your doctor immediately.

Keep the foot elevated on two pillows and wrapped in the elastic bandage. Apply an ice pack over the bandage to the injured ankle, ten minutes on and twenty minutes off, for several hours. Avoid getting the skin wet when icing. Keep the bandage on until the swelling goes down. Applying ice packs to the area of swelling for ten to fifteen minutes three or four times a day is very helpful during recovery.

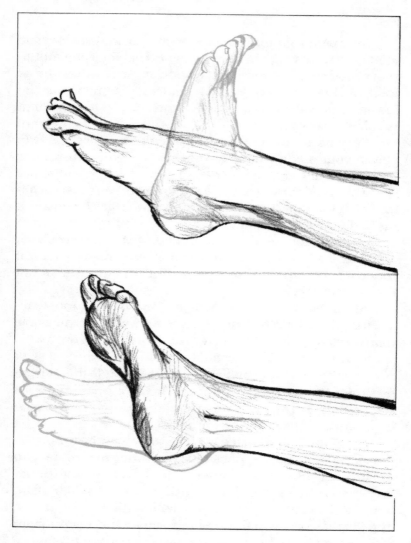

Flex and point exercises are good for an injured ankle.

After the first day, exercise your ankle. You should remove the bandage during exercise and replace it when you're finished. Lie flat on your back, your legs on one or two pillows. Flex your foot toward your face as far as you can move it without pain. Then point your foot away from your face as far as possible. Point your foot away from your face again. Repeat these stretches ten times and do a set two or three times throughout the second day. Keep your foot wrapped in the elastic bandage when you're not exercising and re-wrap it as the swelling goes down. Aspirin is an anti-inflammatory as well as an analgesic and it can help control swelling.

On the third day, add this exercise: lying on your back and holding your foot perpendicular to your leg, turn it inward as far as possible (the right border of your left foot should turn toward the knee, for instance). Repeat ten times, holding the position for a few seconds each time. Then repeat the exercise turning your feet outward as far as you can.

On the third day you can also begin contrast soak therapy. Apply ice for four to six minutes, enough to numb the ankle, then do your flexing exercises and walk on it until you just begin to feel discomfort. Repeat the ice for six to twelve minutes, then stretch and walk again until the pain begins. Ice the ankle a third time.

When you're not icing or exercising your ankle, you should keep it wrapped in the elastic bandage. Repeat the exercise and icing routines daily until you can walk painlessly when you're not wearing the bandage.

When the swelling has disappeared and it no longer hurts to walk, you can resume your normal activities.

Once your ankle is well, however, it's important to

begin strengthening it. You can discontinue your stretching program and start doing isometrics.

Have a friend hold your foot or press it against some object. First press it upward, then press it to the left, to the right and downward. Hold for ten seconds each time. Repeat this cycle five times, two or three times a day for at least a month after your ankle feels well.

You'll know if your ankle has recovered its normal strength by comparing its resistance to the resistance of your healthy ankle as you do this exercise.

When the injured ankle offers as much resistance as the good ankle, you can stop doing your rehabilitation exercises and return to basic stretching.

Of course, if your ankle remains swollen and painful for more than 24 to 48 hours after it is sprained or if it is not feeling better each day using the above therapy, consult your doctor.

MOVING FEET

12

Walking isn't a lost art. One must, by some means,
get out to the garage.
—Evan Esar

A strange coincidence. Many of the symptoms we've long associated with aging—poor circulation, low resistance to infection, brittle bones and weakened muscles—are also the results of being confined to a bed or chair at any age.

The questions among specialists on aging today are: how many of the disabilities we associate with aging are really inevitable and how many could be prevented if we moved our bodies, exercised our muscles and built up our bones?

There's a growing belief among gerontologists that aging doesn't have to be a painful and disabling process.

Yes, some body parts can wear out, and, yes, the body is probably programmed to live a limited number of years. But more and more specialists on aging believe a healthy and productive old age is more normal and natural than the slow deterioration we call aging. But it's no wonder we accept the latter version. Everyone from advertisers and novelists to our doctors and our own children discourages us from doing things. You're too old, they say. Wrinkles are ugly, aging is embarrassing and old people aren't sexy are the messages of our common cultural mythology.

Octogenarian mountain climbers and marathon runners are featured in magazines as freaks of nature, their ages announced in astonishment. How did they do it? We picture ourselves sitting out our retirements in rocking chairs, in lawn chairs or poolside, knitting or reading if our eyes are good or watching youthful types do the real living on daytime soap operas.

Contrary to the Madison Avenue message, the teens and twenties are not the only years to play tennis or water polo, or to sail around the world. Bodies of every age are made to move and moving keeps them healthy. Before we were forced to sit still for more than a decade in school, exercise was fun. Children naturally move around; babies kick until they're strong enough to crawl, crawl until they're strong enough to walk, and walk until they're strong enough to run. Before carriages or cars, people ran everywhere. Muscles that don't move begin to die.

You're never too old to exercise. Each body is constantly rebuilding itself. Your body might heal more slowly with age but it functions the way it always has.

Walking, running and swimming are the best forms of exercise. They're rhythmic and prolonged enough to strengthen your heart and lungs—your cardiovascular system—and they exercise the muscles of your limbs at the same time.

Active muscles massage your insides and stimulate circulation. Moving feet help force the blood back into the heart. Better circulation means better healing powers, more energy and healthier tissues. Exercise helps your body process glucose (simple sugar) more efficiently. It improves your mood, and it keeps bones and muscles strong and flexible. It's the only real wonder drug.

Walking and running are the simplest exercises. You can do them anywhere—the more magnificent the scenery the better—and your only expense is a good pair of shoes.

HOW TO BEGIN

If you have a medical problem or if you are over 40, you should certainly discuss with your physician your exercise program before beginning.

An important thing to consider before you begin your walking or running program is shoes. Good shoes are absolutely essential to prevent injuries and to make moving around fun.

There is nothing more discouraging than launching an exercise program in a pair of shoes that hurt your feet. And there's nothing like your first pair of good running shoes—they're like walking on clouds—to keep your feet safe and happy.

The perfect pair of running shoes has been described as leather with rubber soles. Rubber soles, however, may be hard to find. Most running shoes today are made of

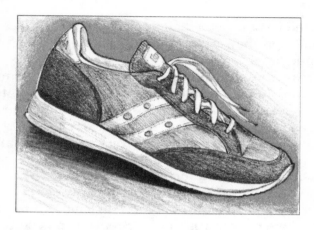

If you are beginning a walking or a running program, a good investment is a well-made pair of running shoes.

synthetics. The soles should be of three layers—a good, sturdy, thick rubber layer in the middle, crepe outer soles and a third layer of cushioning material on the inside.

Leather is the best material for the uppers because it's moldable and adapts to the shape of your foot. As your foot changes size during the day, the leather adapts to it by expanding or contracting. Leather also breathes—it's absorbent and it's good at vaporizing the moisture it absorbs.

Cloth uppers are also good in running and walking shoes because they're light and cool. They will also conform to the shape of your feet. The heel should be sturdy and of a material you can't distort when you press on it with your fingers.

Tennis shoes have low heels and are designed for side to side motion. A running shoe with a heel counter and a heel lift is better for a walking or running program.

GETTING STARTED

Choose a route that's convenient. If you have to drive ten miles to find a place to walk, you'll probably think of lots of reasons to put it off. Choose a spot you love. The more beautiful your route, the more inspired you'll be to do it regularly.

You might want to establish a goal of a certain distance, a mile for example. Or you might just want to walk for a certain period of time, 15 minutes a day for the first week or two, and work slowly up to an hour a day. Walking for a certain amount of time is often more relaxing. You're more likely to pace yourself because you're not trying to cover a fixed distance and get it over with. As a result, you're more likely to enjoy the smells and the sounds and the scenery. You'll be walking this route for a certain amount of time no matter how far it takes you, so you might as well relax and enjoy it.

A good rule of thumb when you're setting your pace while running or walking is to move as quickly as you can while continuing to breathe fairly normally. Naturally, your heart will beat faster and you'll breathe more quickly when you're exerting yourself, but if you're breathing so hard you can't talk, slow down but do not stop. Stopping suddenly puts a strain on the cardiovascular system. Check your pulse while continuing to walk. Your maximum pulse rate should be 220 minus your age. For example, if you're 55, your maximum pulse rate is 165. Your training pulse rate is between 70 and 80 percent of the maximum. That is between 116 and 132 if you're 55. Over 132 puts a strain on the cardiovascular system. Below 116 does not benefit your heart. Learn to monitor your pulse as you walk and run.

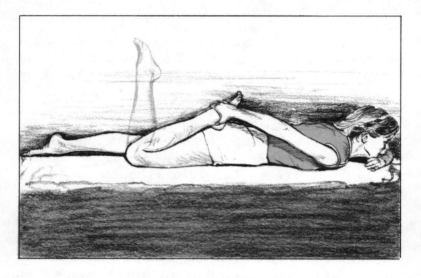

Stretch quadriceps by gently pulling your ankle toward your but-
tocks. Alternate legs, three times each.

Always stretch for ten minutes before and after you
exercise. Here are four good stretches you can do.

To loosen your quadriceps (the long muscles on the
front of your thighs), lie face down on the floor or ground
and bend one leg, pulling your ankle toward your buttocks
until you can feel the stretch in your quadriceps. If it
hurts, you're stretching it too far. Hold the stretch for 20
seconds, then relax and stretch the other leg for 20 seconds. Stretch each leg three times. Simultaneously contract the muscles on the back of your leg for a safer
stretch.

To limber up your calf muscles, stand with your arms
extended in front of you, your hands pressed against a

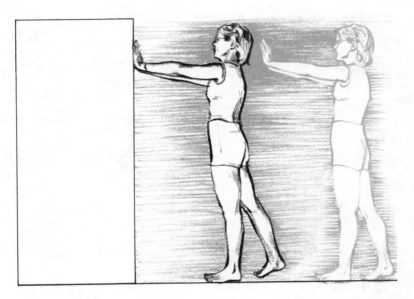

Loosen calf muscles by pressing your extended heel toward the floor. Feel the stretch in the mid-calf area.

door or wall and your feet flat against the floor. Extend one foot behind you, the other foot still flat on the floor and perpendicular to the wall. You must keep your knee straight and not hyperextend your back. Gently press the heel of the extended foot toward the floor until you can feel the pull in the muscle in the middle of your calf. Hold each leg in this position for 20 seconds and repeat three times.

For your hamstrings (the muscles in the backs of your thighs), lie flat on your back and lift one leg into the air. With your knee just slightly bent, use a towel to pull your leg toward you until you can feel the stretch in the middle

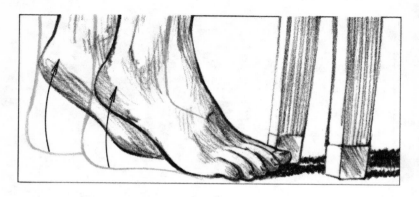

Raising yourself on your toes and gently lowering will help strengthen calf muscles.

of the back of your thigh. Hold the stretch for 20 seconds and do it three times with each leg.

To strengthen the calf muscles, hold the back of a chair for balance and raise yourself up on your toes. Do this five times, holding the stretch for ten seconds each time. Always hold these stretches gently and never bounce. Bouncing is counterproductive because it irritates the muscle and forces it to contract.

If you feel any soreness in your knees or feet after your run or walk, ice the sore spots immediately to prevent any irritation from becoming an injury. You can use ice cubes in a plastic bag. Rub this cold pack on the irritation.

Another way to apply ice is to fill a styrofoam cup ¾ full of water. Freeze it. Then cut the bottom and an inch of the side off. Massage the area with the ice using the styrofoam as a handle.

EXERCISE YOUR FEET

13

When I was 40, my doctor advised me that a man in his forties shouldn't play tennis. I heeded his advice carefully and could hardly wait until I reached 50 to start again.
—Justice Hugo Black as quoted in Think, *February, 1963*

Many muscles, tendons and ligaments connect the 26 bones and many joints in each of your feet. If any of these parts fails, your foot is thrown out of balance and the other parts must compensate.

Balance means that each muscle group is equally as strong as its opposing muscle group so that your muscles can contract, stretch and relax. If any muscle or tendon becomes tighter or more developed than its opposite, the whole system changes and your bones are pulled into a different position.

91

The best way to enhance muscle balance is to stretch and exercise. Stretching should be done daily. The more perfectly your bones and connective tissue are aligned, the more flexible and strong your feet and ankles will be. Strong, flexible feet are less vulnerable to injury.

Remember to exercise gently. Never work a muscle until it hurts and don't work out to the point of exhaustion. If you start with just a single repetition today, you might be able to do each exercise three or four times tomorrow or the next day. So establish a reasonable goal and work up to it slowly.

Foot exercises may be done barefoot or in sturdy running shoes.

Vigorously shake out your feet for a full minute before you exercise them to relax muscles and to warm them up.

Standing Foot Stretch
This is a very simple exercise and you should do this for a few days if the others are too painful at first.

1) Stand facing a wall, hands at chest level. Your feet should be parallel and six inches apart.
2) Tuck your buttocks down to elongate your waist. Stand up straight pushing up through the top of your head, keeping your chin down. Tense your thighs and keep your knees facing forward. Spread your toes, and then relax them.
3) Inhale and lift your heels, rising onto the balls of your feet. Have a friend watch you and make sure your heels are aligned with your toes. Hold the position for ten seconds or as long as you can.
4) Exhale and descend slowly to your heels. Be sure your toes are relaxed.

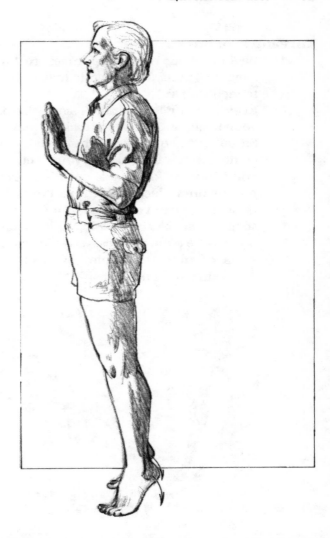

The Standing Foot Stretch is a simple exercise which strengthens the back of the leg and inner foot muscles.

Kneeling Foot Stretch

1) Begin on your hands and knees, resting the weight of your feet on your toes which are turned under.

2) Keeping your feet parallel, slowly sit back on your heels until your buttocks touch your feet. Sit tall but allow the weight of your body to gently stretch the soles of your feet.

   You can wear knee pads or do this exercise on a mat or on a piece of foam you've spread on the floor to protect your knees. Of course, common sense must be used in doing this and all exercises. If you have pain, stiffness, swelling, and any other signs of muscle or joint overuse, discontinue exercising and take a rest.

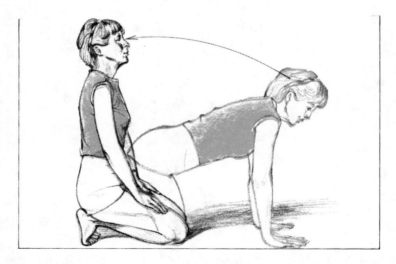

The Kneeling Foot Stretch will stretch the soles of your feet and take stress off your back.

Foot Extensions

1) Lie on your back, arms at your sides, with both knees bent and your feet flat on the floor. Bring one knee to your chest, exhale, and lift your foot into the air. Your knee can be slightly bent.

2) Bend your foot at the ankle and flex it toward the front of your leg, pushing out on your heel. Spread your toes.

3) Push out on the ball of the foot, bending your foot at the ankle toward the back of your leg, but keep your toes flexed toward your knee.

4) Finally, point the toes as a ballet dancer would, squeezing ("wrinkling") the sole of the foot and feeling the stretch in the front of the ankle and foot.

5) Reverse the three actions, moving slowly from one position to the other. Repeat the sequence using your other foot.

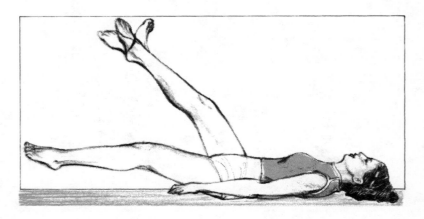

Foot Extensions are good for front and back muscles of lower leg.

Toe Stretch

You can do this sitting in a chair or lying on your back. Spread your toes as far apart as you can. Hold for five seconds if you can. Relax. Curl your toes for five seconds. Relax and repeat. At the first sign of cramps, immediately stretch in the opposite direction and begin massaging the area.

Walking on Your Toes

Practice walking around on your toes. You can do this either as a part of your exercise routine or just walking around the house when you think of it. It's a great way to stretch and strengthen your feet.

Foot Press

Sitting on a chair or the edge of your bed, put one foot on top of the other and press them against one another,

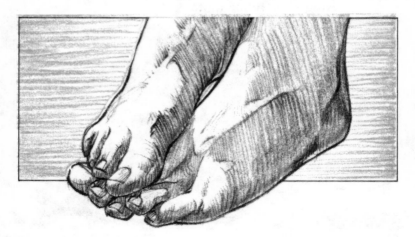

You can do the foot press exercise while reading or watching TV.

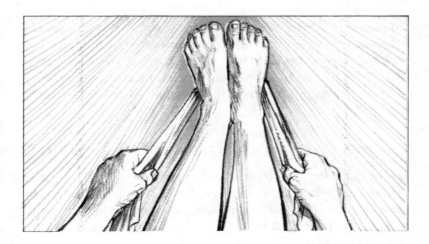

The towel pull is a good isometric exercise.

pushing up with the lower foot and down with the foot on top. Hold this press for ten to fifteen seconds and do it again with the feet in opposite positions.

Towel Pull
Still sitting, take the ends of a towel in your hands and put it under your feet like a sling. Use it to pull your feet toward you while you're pushing against it with your feet. Hold this for ten to fifteen seconds, relax and repeat. Both the foot press and this exercise are good isometric exercises to strengthen your feet.

EXERCISE TO STRENGTHEN WEAK ARCHES

If your feet hurt during the day or your soles seem to burn, your longitudinal arches are probably caving in due to constant strain. It is difficult to strengthen a weak arch. The simple exercises just recommended can help. Toe curling, stretching, and foot rotation are particularly helpful. Once the arches are weak or collapsed, however, they need external support from proper shoes or orthotic devices.

OTHER GOOD EXERCISES FOR YOUR FEET

Jumping rope is a great way to strengthen your feet and ankles and you can do it anywhere. It's also a good cardiovascular exercise and, like any exercise program, should be preceded by a physical exam and consultation with your doctor.

The best overall foot exercise, though, is walking. You can practice for your walks indoors. As you move around your house or apartment, be sure you're walking properly. Your heel should hit the ground first, your weight rolling quickly to your toe. Ideally your feet should be nearly parallel or turned out no more than 15°. Have a friend watch to find out if you're doing it properly.

When you can't walk, passive exercises like massage and manipulation of your feet and legs by a therapist also help improve circulation and generally stimulate the tissue in your feet.

EXERCISES TO DO IN A CHAIR

You can do these exercises at your desk or in a chair while you're reading, talking or watching TV.

1) First limber your foot by simply rotating it at the ankle.

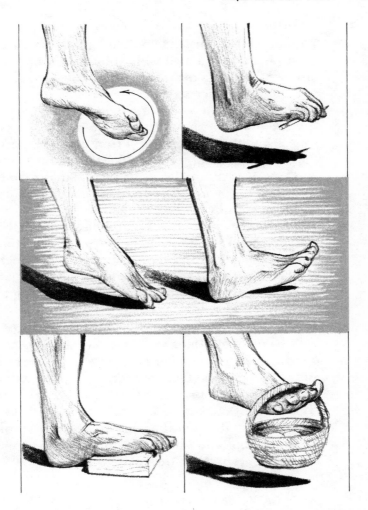

You can perform some foot exercises while sitting: top, rotate the ankle; pick up objects with the toes; center, tap toe and heel to the floor; bottom, stand on a wedge and lift small weights with your feet.

2)   To tone your ligaments and tendons, try picking up a pencil or a towel with your toes. Don't be discouraged if it's difficult at first. With practice, you'll find it easier to do.

3)   Stretch your leg tendons (the tendons running up the back of your ankle from your heel) and calf muscles with this exercise. From a sitting position, alternately tap on the floor with your heels and toes. You should feel a gentle pull in the front of your leg as you tap your toe, a gentle pull up the back of your heel as you tap your heel.

4)   You can also stretch your Achilles tendon by standing with your heels on the floor and your toes on a block of wood or a "flex-wedge" which can be adjusted for various angles of stretch. Like all stretches, this should pull gently and should never hurt.

5)   Finish your exercise routine by lifting weights with your feet. Hang a purse or some other weight from your ankle and lift your leg while sitting. You should feel the exertion in the center of your quadriceps, the muscle in the front of your thigh. Don't try to lift something that's too heavy to do this comfortably. You want some resistance but you don't want to strain the muscle. Don't completely extend your knee.

EXERCISES TO DO IN BED

If you're confined to your bed or even if you have a hard time getting started in the morning, these warm-up exercises for your feet can be done both before you get out of bed in the morning and before you fall asleep at night.

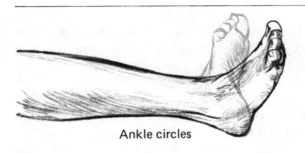

Ankle circles

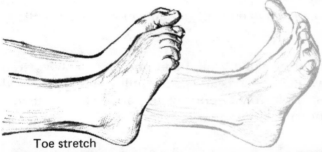

Toe stretch

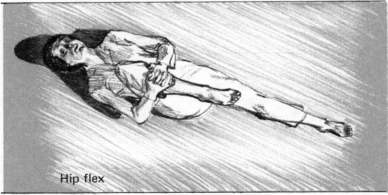

Hip flex

Some exercises can be done in while lying in bed: top, *ankle circles;* center, *toe stretch;* bottom, *hip flex.*

Toe Stretch

Lying on your back, curl your toes and hold for a count of ten. Then bend your toes slowly back, spreading them at the same time. Hold again for a count of ten.

Ankle Circles

First, turn your right foot in a counter-clockwise direction, rotating it at the ankle. (Be sure all the motion is in the ankle, not in the knees or hips.) Do it slowly and deliberately.

Second, rotate your left foot in a clockwise direction.

Hip Flex

Still lying flat on your back, bend one knee slowly. Grab your leg with both hands and gently pull your knee toward your chest. Hold for a count of ten and release. Repeat with the other leg.

DIABETES AND YOUR FEET

14

Man may be the captain of his fate,
but he is also the victim of his blood sugar.
—*Wilfrid G. Oakley,* Transactions of the
Medical Society of London, 1962

Infections that don't heal, poor circulation and numbness in your feet are some of the secondary effects of diabetes, a disease characterized by faulty sugar metabolism. Because an infection that doesn't heal can lead to serious complications (gangrene, for instance, is the death of the deep tissue in the area of the infection), it's especially important that diabetics prevent infections with careful foot care.

Poor sugar metabolism will affect circulation, and feet usually show the first symptoms of poor circulation because they're farthest from the heart. Your feet might develop ulcers that don't heal, brittle nails, dry skin, tingling and even numbness when the arteries narrow, starving peripheral nerves and causing permanent damage.

DIABETES DO'S AND DON'TS

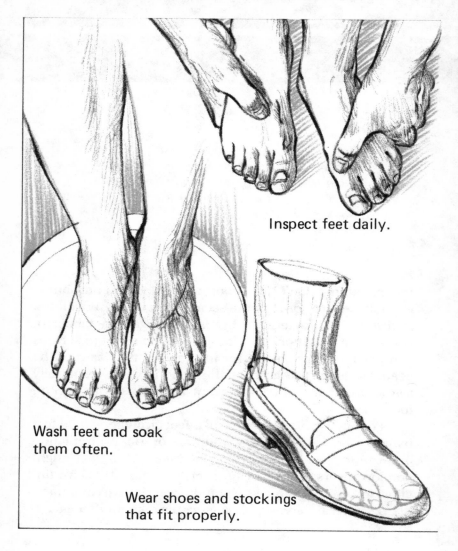

Inspect feet daily.

Wash feet and soak them often.

Wear shoes and stockings that fit properly.

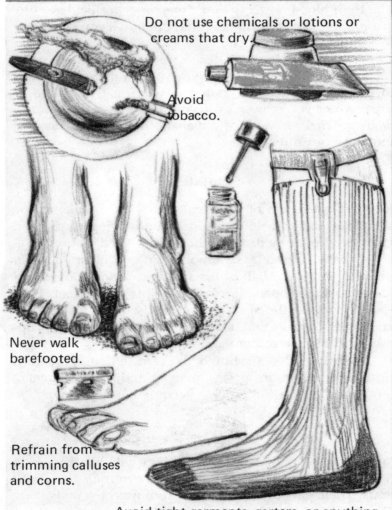

Do not use chemicals or lotions or creams that dry.

Avoid tobacco.

Never walk barefooted.

Refrain from trimming calluses and corns.

Avoid tight garments, garters, or anything that will restrict circulation.

High blood sugar makes the skin a perfect breeding ground for bacteria, a dangerous situation if you can't even feel injuries to your feet.

Women develop diabetes more frequently than men. If you're a middle-aged adult, you're ten times more likely to develop this disease than you were at twenty-five or thirty. Once you're over sixty, your chances of becoming a diabetic triple. If you are a diabetic patient, professional foot care is a must.

ULCERS

An early symptom of diabetes, ulcers are breaks in the skin that cause disintegration of underlying tissue and grow progressively deeper when not treated.

Usually caused by irritation or injury, ulcers develop most often on the ball of the foot because of foot imbalance causing abnormal pressure points on the feet. They also develop at the sites of neglected corns and calluses and under toenails that have either been trimmed improperly or subjected to tight shoes.

Diabetic ulcers should be treated immediately. Untreated ulcers are easily infected and, in the diabetic foot, an infection can quickly become life-threatening.

INCURVATED NAILS

Another result of diabetes and other circulatory disorders, incurvated nails are among the most common nail problems. Their effect is similar to that of ingrown nails; they grow into the toe's soft tissue and cause a great deal of pain if cut improperly.

Incurvated nails can't be prevented by cutting your toenails properly. Caused by an inadequate blood supply to the nail bed, the sides of these nails actually begin to curve down into the skin and the undernourished skin may begin to thicken.

Eventually, these nails may need to be removed. Less radical treatment isn't always effective because the problem is the inadequate blood supply and, if it isn't corrected, the nail will continue to emerge distorted. Always have your podiatrist trim these nails; it's dangerous to attempt trimming them yourself.

CARING FOR DIABETIC FEET

If you are a diabetic, there are certain cautions you should observe:

- See your podiatrist at least once a month. You should always have your podiatrist trim your nails because an ingrown nail or even the slightest nick in the skin from nail scissors can cause a serious infection. If your nails are brittle, you can soak and cream them at home, but don't try to cut them yourself. And never try to treat the simplest foot problem, even a corn or callus, on your own.

- Don't use any over-the-counter medications on your feet (corn or callus medications or antiseptics, for example) unless they are prescribed for you. They can cause ulcers on the feet even if you don't have circulatory problems.

- Wash your feet daily with soap and warm (never hot) water. Gently pat them dry with a towel paying special attention to the area between your toes. Use a lotion to massage your feet morning and night to keep the skin soft. You can use a lanolin-based moisturizer or body cream.

- Don't walk barefoot. It's easy to step on splinters and, if you've lost sensation in your feet, you won't feel them. Inspect your feet daily for any injuries or abnormalities.

- Wear only soft leather or cloth shoes. Shoes made of reptile skin, plastic or patent leather aren't porous or flexible enough. Your shoes should fit with no points of irritation. Never wear constricting boots. Women's high, tight-legged boots can cause circulatory problems even in otherwise healthy feet.

- Don't use circular garters or wear socks with a tight top band. Don't wear support hose unless prescribed; you don't need anything constricting your feet and inhibiting circulation. Be sure your socks fit comfortably; be careful that the rough edges of a mended sock don't irritate your feet.

- If your feet perspire excessively, ask your podiatrist or family doctor to prescribe a safe foot powder or soak.

- Get plenty of exercise to stimulate circulation and don't smoke or drink coffee. Nicotine and caffeine impair circulation.

FOOT SURGERY

15

"The sensation of being cut by a skilful surgeon would not, I think, be pain, if one could keep one's imagination out of it." —J.A. Spender, The Comments of Bagshot.

Foot surgery is most commonly elective surgery. In other words, unless your foot must be treated for an infection and trauma or amputated because of spreading gangrene, foot surgery is not a life and death matter. It's a matter of your choice.

In treating older people, many doctors have traditionally balanced the risk of surgery against a patient's life expectancy. If you were eighty and developing bunions, for example, certain types of foot surgery might be ruled out on the grounds that surgery was too risky. "We have been conditioned to think about surgery in terms of young and middle-aged adults," writes one podiatrist in a medical school textbook.

Fortunately, even doctors are beginning to understand that average life expectancy has nothing to do with your personal life expectancy. An average life expectancy of seventy can mean you'll live to be forty-five or ninety-five.

And when you're ninety-five, mobility is more important than it was when you were fifteen. Mobility means independence; losing it usually means a decline in physical and mental health.

If you have a foot problem that's painful and debilitating and less radical treatment hasn't helped, you'll probably consider surgery.

It's important that you discuss the benefits and risks of surgery with the doctor that recommends it. Follow the advice of the person in whom you have the most confidence.

WHEN FOOT SURGERY CAN HELP

Surgery can be very useful when other treatments fail to change your condition.

Surgery can correct chronic ingrown toenails, corns and severe calluses. When heel spurs are painfully crippling and *steroid injections don't offer relief,* they can be removed. If some of your toes have protruding bones that irritate the other toes, perhaps causing chronic soft corns, the bones can be realigned or the protruberances removed, often on an ambulatory out-patient basis.

Surgery can correct toes that overlap or underlap or toes that are contracted, as in hammertoes. Neuromas (nerves trapped or pinched as the result of pressure on the foot) are often surgically removed. Swollen bursas (the fluid-filled sacs that overlay the joints) and painful bunions can also be surgically corrected.

TOENAIL SURGERY

Ingrown toenails are the most common cause of pain in the aging foot. If the nail has been ingrown for some time, is infected and deeply imbedded in the soft tissues on either or both sides of the nail, your podiatrist will need to remove the irritating corner of the nail, along with some of the soft tissue, in order to treat the infection.

If you're an uncontrolled diabetic or have a circulatory problem, your resistance to infection is lower than normal, and your toes don't have the circulation of blood necessary to heal surgical wounds quickly, so your podiatrist probably will try to avoid cutting into tissue. He or she might opt instead to remove the entire nail being careful to avoid cutting the nail bed and the soft tissue on either side of the nail. Free of the irritating nail, the infected soft tissue has a chance to heal and a new nail will grow in. As the new nail comes in, your podiatrist should inspect it regularly. This can take as long as six months to a year or more to heal.

AMBULATORY VERSUS TRADITIONAL SURGERY

The purpose of surgery should be to eliminate the pain in your foot and to restore as much mobility as possible. The procedure should be simple and direct.

There is some controversy as to how simple and direct surgery to reconstruct bones and tendons should be.

Foot surgery is commonly performed by both podiatrists and orthopedic surgeons. Both have a four-year medical school background and post-graduate surgical training ranging from one to five years.

Ambulatory surgery seems to offer substantial advantages. A long recovery period can be dangerous as you grow older. It increases the chances of postoperative complications like pneumonia and blood clots. The sooner you're walking around, the sooner your wound can heal and the less opportunity your muscles will have to atrophy from disuse. Ambulatory surgery can be performed with a general anesthetic or a local anesthetic block.

Preparing for Surgery

Discuss the goals of surgery with your foot specialist. Sometimes the purpose of surgery is to prevent a condition from getting worse, rather than to improve it, and it's best if you and your doctor agree on the goals of your operation.

Your doctor will probably run a series of lab tests to make sure you're healthy enough to undergo an operation safely. Tests might include a foot X ray, a urinalysis and a series of blood and liver tests. If the operation involves general anesthesia, you'll be given an electrocardiogram and a chest X ray.

Surgery should be put off:

- If your podiatrist recommends it,
- If you have or are recovering from an upper respiratory tract infection,
- If you're taking digitalis for a heart condition and are showing any signs of digitalis poisoning because your kidneys aren't functioning adequately,

- If you're taking diuretics for a heart condition or hypertension and they've affected your blood volume or electrolyte balance,
- If you're diabetic and your circulation is inadequate and/or your hyperglycemia is not under control,
- If, for any reason, circulation to your feet is inadequate,
- If, because of poor diet or an illness, you're suffering from malnutrition,
- If you're recovering from a recent heart attack.

All of these should be discussed with your doctor or surgeon before any decision is made.

Ask your doctor to explain the operation and to tell you what will be expected of you when it's over. Do this before the operation.

Most foot surgery can be completed in less than an hour. The simpler the surgical procedure, the less likely it will be followed by a long recovery period. Extensive bed rest after an operation can undo all the good effected by the surgery.

You should be well-nourished and drink plenty of water in the weeks before surgery. If you're showing symptoms of malnutrition or dehydration, your foot specialist will probably put off the procedure until you've had an opportunity to make up these deficiencies.

Your doctor might put you on a diet high in protein with iron and vitamin supplements. A vitamin C deficiency can delay healing, and lack of any of the B-complex vitamins can inhibit your body's ability to use carbohydrates and protein.

AFTER SURGERY

It's important, especially when you're older and vulnerable to so many postoperative complications, that you be properly cared for when surgery is over.

Venous thrombosis or the formation of blood clots in your veins is one of the most serious postoperative complications that can affect older people. To stimulate circulation and prevent blood clots, your doctor will probably apply compression bandages to your feet to stimulate blood flow and to control postoperative swelling, which can inhibit circulation.

Immediately after surgery, your doctor will probably try to make you cough and will prescribe exercises to aerate your lungs and prevent pneumonia.

As soon as you can after surgery, and your surgeon allows, you should start moving and then walking.

You should take your temperature regularly while you're recovering from any operation. Taking it once in the morning and once before you go to bed will alert you to a change in temperature that might signify a postoperative problem.

Ask your foot surgeon how often you should clean and change the dressing on your wound.

Most important after surgery is regular contact with your foot surgeon, especially if you notice continued pain and any special weakness, fever or another change in your physical condition.

IS SURGERY REALLY NECESSARY?

Take your time. Be wary of any foot surgeon who insists on immediate surgery for any condition short of a serious infection or threat of life or limb. Foot surgery is rarely an emergency. You must have confidence in your doctor's recommendations before proceeding with surgery.

Be wary of doctors who act as if you've asked them their sexual preferences when you ask about fees. For too long there's been a sort of taboo about discussing money with doctors, as if it weren't quite polite, until it becomes a matter of paying the bill.

It's not necessary that you choose the cheapest service—in medicine, as in other things, you often get what you pay for. But it's good to know if your doctor's fees are in line with the fees of his or her peers. If they're not, you have every right to know why. The important thing is to know what you're being offered for your money.

16

KNOW YOUR MEDICATION

When it comes to your health, I recommend frequent doses of that rare commodity among Americans—common sense.
—Dr. Vincent Askey, speech to a medical convention, Bakersfield, California 1960

The aspirin you take to reduce the pain and swelling in your big toe joint does not stop there. Unfortunately it circulates throughout your system. Every medication has side effects, and as you take more, the effects become more complicated. Some drugs heighten the effects of others, some inhibit or completely counteract the effects of another and others form combinations that can harm or even kill you. According to one recent medical text, the incidence of adverse reactions while taking one to five drugs is 18.6 percent. With six or more drugs, the number of incidents soars to 81.4 percent.

Multiple daily doses of medications and vitamins may be necessary, though. You might be suffering from more than one disease or from vitamin deficiency. Often vitamins are needed to supplement your medication because some medicines impede your body's ability to use nutrients in the food you eat.

Drug interactions can be dangerous. Even the minor effects of mixing drugs can have serious consequences. Suppose your doctor prescribes a drug to control your high blood pressure. The medicine makes your nose stuffy so you take an over-the-counter decongestant without telling your doctor. One of the side effects of most decongestants is to increase your blood pressure. When your doctor discovers the increase, he or she decides your dosage of the high-blood-pressure medicine isn't high enough and increases it.

Drugs can also mask the symptoms of an illness. Medicine may relieve the pain, for example, while the illness continues unnoticed and perhaps with additional harm to your body. For example, you can mask the symptoms of arthritis by taking aspirin or of a peptic ulcer by taking antacids. Then the arthritis or ulcer continues to do harm while you are ignoring it because you have no pain. To avoid masking the symptoms of serious problems, never take an over-the-counter medicine for more than a few days without checking with your doctor.

Your body's response to a drug can change as you grow older as well. For instance, poor kidney and liver function can render a normally therapeutic dose toxic. Also, as you grow older, the muscle/fat ratio changes and affects your response to drugs. Your diet, your emotional state, your weight and your health can all determine how you'll respond to a drug.

The most reliable source of information on the effects of drugs on your body is you. You're the only person who knows how many doctors you're seeing, what they've prescribed, how often you take the drugs and what, if any, strange effects medicine has had on you in the past. Tell your doctor about all prescription and over-the-counter drugs you're taking. You may find it helpful to make a list and carry it with you. Describe any peculiar side-effects or adverse reactions you've had to a drug and ask questions. It's important that you understand exactly what your doctor is prescribing. What are the side effects? What are the risks? What is the effect of combining this drug with other medicines you're taking? Are there any over-the-counter drugs that can affect or be affected by the action of this new prescription?

NUTRITION AND DRUGS

Even the famous father of medicine, Hippocrates (460 to 370 B.C.), said diet was a crucial part of medical therapy.

Many of the problems associated with aging are actually the results of long-term dietary deficiencies. With age, the body burns energy more slowly. Digestion can be inhibited if stomach acid production declines and the stomach wall loses its tone. As muscles lose tone from the inactivity that often accompanies aging in our culture, the emptying of the stomach and the movement of the bowels slows down. Circulation can also be inhibited and nourishment to blood-fed body parts cut off.

If you're missing some teeth, if you've lost some of your ability to taste or smell, or if your coordination is somehow impaired so that using a knife and fork seems more trouble than it's worth, you might lose your motivation to eat.

A lifetime of poor eating habits eventually catches up with you. Even if you're eating the way you always did (sometimes especially if you're eating the way you always did), the results of deficiencies in your diet begin to take their toll.

Drugs taken to control the effects of aging can cause further nutritional deficiencies by inhibiting the absorption of vitamins and minerals. Certain foods, on the other hand, may inhibit the effects of your medication. Discuss with your doctor if you should take your medication with certain foods or if there are some foods you should avoid.

BUYING MEDICATION

The sheer number of medicines, the multitude of new drugs that flood the market every year and differences in labeling, all conspire to make a mystery of the drug world.

Find a pharmacist who is willing to take the time to explain what you're buying and how effective it is, a pharmacist who is familiar with the strengths and weaknesses of different drug manufacturers.

Be sure you understand when you should take the drug (before or after a meal), how you should take it (with or without milk or water), how often you should take it and for how long you should take it.

Recent studies also show that half of us don't follow the directions that come with prescription drugs. If you take a lot of medicine, ask for written instructions from your doctor and be sure you understand them. Use a calendar to keep track of the times you take your medicine

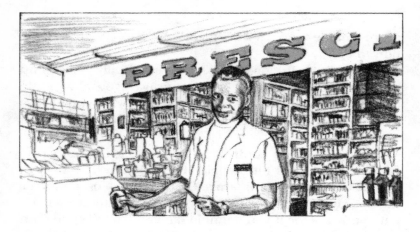

Find a pharmacist who will take time to discuss your medications.

or collect the day's pills in a separate vial so you'll remember which ones you've taken.

Most important, be sure you know the names of all the drugs you're taking and whether or not they can be mixed with over-the-counter medicines, with alcohol or with the other drugs you're taking.

OVER-THE-COUNTER MEDICINES FOR THE FOOT

Pain Relief

There's probably no drug more popular than aspirin for relieving pain. Aspirin, taken in large doses under the supervision of your doctor, is also effective in relieving joint inflammation, and arthritics are usually encouraged to take at least six aspirin a day depending on the severity of their condition.

Not everyone can take aspirin. If you have allergies and aren't sure how you'll react to aspirin, avoid taking it. If you have diabetes, take aspirin cautiously, and if you have peptic ulcers or a bleeding problem, don't take it at all.

Aspirin is often found in products that contain other drugs. Some are made in combination with antacids; others contain additional pain relivers or caffeine.

You might want to use a buffered aspirin to protect your stomach lining. Some combination or coated products help reduce stomach irritation because they dissolve in the intestine rather than in the stomach.

Another effective over-the-counter pain reliever is acetaminophen, an aspirin-free pain reliever. Acetaminophen doesn't upset the stomach or interfere with blood clotting as aspirin does, but it's also less effective in relieving pain, especially pain associated with redness or swelling. If you have a headache and an upset stomach, take acetaminophen. But if you want relief from swollen joints, aspirin is best.

There is an endless number of products marketed to be applied directly to your skin to relieve muscle pain. These drugs, called external analgesics (pain relievers) all act as counter-irritants, relieving pain by increasing the flow of blood to the muscle and producing warmth, and irritating the skin to override the pain sensation.

Although some contain a dizzying number of ingredients, they all usually contain a heat-generating substance like methyl salicylate (wintergreen oil), mustard oil, turpentine oil or camphor. Products with wintergreen oil must be rubbed in well and are probably most effective because the massaging is as likely to relieve soreness as is the product. Never apply these ointments to broken skin, to mucous membranes or to inflamed areas. Wash your hands well after using them because even a little rubbed accidentally in your eyes can be extremely irritating. You may even want to wear rubber gloves while applying it.

Remember that the effects of these analgesics are temporary. If you have muscle pain for more than a few days, you should consult with your doctor.

Anti-bacterial and Anti-fungal Medicines

Anti-infectives are anti-bacterial medicines used to prevent infection from cuts and abrasions. Applying an anti-infective to a cut or abrasion is not usually necessary; you can usually prevent infection by simply washing the wound well with a mild soap and water or with hydrogen peroxide.

Seventy percent ethyl rubbing alcohol is effective as an anti-infective for only a short time. Mercurochrome is not only irritating to open cuts but is also fairly useless as an anti-infective. Stains like gentian violet and scarlet red are effective as both anti-bacterial and anti-fungal agents superficially. Their main drawback is that they're messy and tend to obscure the wound, making it difficult to treat. Some topical creams and ointments are also usually very effective in fighting bacteria. The disadvantage of ointments is that they are absorbed too well and tend to coat the skin and prevent moisture from entering or escaping the site of application. For this reason, they aren't recommended for use between your toes where trapped moisture can cause fungal infections.

Tolnaftate is the most popular and effective anti-fungal ("athlete's foot") agent. It's a relatively safe drug.

Toxic reactions are rare and mild. You can buy it in cream, liquid, powder and aerosol powder forms. Look for it as an ingredient in athlete's foot remedies.

Moisturizers
Dry skin is a frequent problem in aging feet, especially feet with poor circulation.

Avoid products like petroleum jellies that feel greasy and tend to coat and moisture-proof your skin. These can trap moisture on the surface of your skin and cause fungal infections, especially between your toes.

A ten or twenty percent urea cream that can be applied after washing or soaking your feet is an excellent moisturizer.

Zinc oxide ointment is great for protecting moist sores and cuts. It also absorbs moisture so it helps protect the affected area from friction and infection. The zinc is a mild tissue stimulant.

Wart, Corn and Callus Removers
Avoid corn, callus and wart removers unless prescribed by your podiatrist. Most of them contain products like salicylic acid, acetic acid or zinc chloride that are highly corrosive. They work by dissolving the tissue of the corn, wart, or callus, but they don't, unfortunately, distinguish between healthy and dead tissue.

PRESCRIPTION DRUGS

Antibiotics
An oral antibiotic medicine used to treat a foot infection can be inhibited by poor circulation. If your circulation is

impaired, your doctor may need to prescribe a higher-than-normal dose.

Some foods prevent oral antibiotics from working effectively. Tetracycline, for example, is inactivated by milk products and antacids. Ask your doctor or pharmacist for specific advice on taking antibiotics.

Anti-inflammatory Agents (Nonsteroid)

Indomethacin is used for short-term inflammatory conditions like heel bursitis, acute gouty arthritis, rheumatoid arthritis, and osteoarthritis. It can upset your stomach so it must be taken after a meal, with food, or with milk or an antacid. Aspirin inhibits the effects of this drug.

Ibuprofen is a newer anti-inflammatory drug that is somewhat safer than indomethacin. Ibuprofen, too, should be taken with milk or a meal and should not be taken with aspirin.

Uricosurics help your body rid itself of uric acid through the urine and are used to treat gout. They can't relieve gouty attacks but they can prevent them.

Steroids

Steroids are the most widely used injectable and oral drugs. They are excellent anti-inflammatory agents and are used to reduce swelling in all types of tissue.

Steroids are a group of hormones produced by adrenal glands or synthetically in laboratories. They reduce inflammatory, allergic and rheumatic reactions and are therefore referred to as anti-inflammatory hormones, as corticosteroids or as glucocorticoids.

Steroids also affect sugar, protein and calcium metabolism and this function sometimes limits their effectiveness as therapeutic agents. Taken in large doses over an extended period of time, they can cause salt and water retention and potassium loss, high blood sugar, osteoporosis or weakened bones, slower healing of wounds, impaired fat metabolism, impaired calcium excretion and kidney stones. They can lower your resistance to infection and they can cause mood changes.

Steroids come in many different forms, each designed to maximize the therapeutic effects on certain tissues and to minimize the less desirable effects.

Soaks

A Burow's solution soak is used as an astringent soak. A dissolving tablet or powder, it is a good astringent that also acts as an anti-fungal agent. Used on foot ulcers, open fissures or after nail surgery, it keeps the foot clean.

Epsom salts in solution help relieve swelling and are generally refreshing. They can be purchased without a prescription. Also, a tablespoon of salt in a quart of lukewarm water is a soothing, inexpensive soak.

Antifungal Agents

Haloprogin and Clotrimazole are available as creams and liquids and are very effective in treating foot fungus infections.

SUMMARY: WHEN YOU'RE TAKING MEDICATION

- Always know the name of the drug and its effects, both therapeutic and adverse.
- Be sure your doctor knows what other drugs, both over-the-counter and prescription, you're

taking when he or she prescribes a new medication.

- Be sure you understand when you should take a drug, how you should take it (with or without milk, before or after a meal), and for how long you should take it.
- Ask your doctor about the effects of mixing it with other drugs you normally ingest, whether they be aspirin, multi-vitamins, alcohol or marijuana.
- Develop a good relationship with your pharmacist. Choose a pharmacist who is willing to discuss the benefits and cost-savings of different brand names and generic versions of the medicines you're taking.
- Buy only as much of a drug as you need. Drugs lose their effectiveness after a certain period of time. Know the shelf-life of your drugs.
- Keep your drug intake to a minimum. Remember that the adverse effects of mixing drugs soar when you're taking more than one drug.
- Keep up your knowledge of medications you are taking. The AARP Pharmacy Service offers an easily available source of information on vitamins and other medication.

PHYSICAL THERAPY

17

*I enjoy convalescence. It is the
part that makes the illness worthwhile.*
—*George Bernard Shaw,* Back to Methuselah

If you're recovering from surgery or another foot ailment, if your feet are stiff and aching with arthritis or if you're suffering the effects of poor circulation, the most important and effective treatment is to actively rehabilitate your foot. Drugs and surgery can relieve pain and sometimes remove the condition that's causing it, but they can't restore your foot's full function without active physical therapy.

Exercise is the most effective physical therapy. It limbers and strengthens muscles and tendons and it thickens bones, but passive therapies—massage, soaks and the application of heat, sound and electrical currents—can all help speed healing when properly used.

THERMOTHERAPY—HEAT AND COLD

Cryotherapy (Ice Packs)

Because heat increases skin surface temperature and can encourage blood to pool and swelling to increase, you'll want to apply ice to any injury or surgical wound for the first two or three days. Ice reduces swelling and prevents blood from pooling in the injured area.

You can freeze water in five-ounce cups. Place that or an ice cube in a plastic bag and cover with a dry towel. Rub the covered ice in a circular motion on the injury for five to ten minutes per hour. Ice as frequently as you can in the first few days after an injury. Do not use ice on a fresh wound. Icing can be especially effective when it's alternated with gentle stretching exercises. Never strap or tape the ice to your body. To do so can cause serious skin damage similar to frostbite.

Whirlpools

Whether you have a painful, disabling condition like arthritis or you've injured yourself and have been icing the injury for several days, whirlpools are a great way to gently massage and soothe sore joints or muscles to speed healing.

Letting your foot rest passively in a pool of warm water, though, can make it swell as the blood begins to pool around the heated area. You should exercise your foot to prevent swelling. You can do some of the exercises described in Chapter 13. You needn't do them quickly or vigorously; just keep your feet moving.

You can soak your feet in a whirlpool as often as you like. The water temperature should be 93 to 102 degrees if only your foot is submerged. (It should be less than 97 degrees if your whole body is submerged.) Be sure you're not cutting off circulation by rolling up your pants or by resting your legs on the rim of the tub.

Hot Compresses
You can apply a hot compress (a hot water bottle wrapped in a towel or a heating pad are safest and most effective) for ten to thirty minutes two or three times a day to soothe aching joints and to heal injured muscles.

Be careful, though. If you have any problems with circulation or sensations in your feet that have made it more difficult for you to feel heat or cold, don't apply heat yourself because you'll have no way of knowing whether you're burning yourself.

And never, never fall asleep with a heating pad. The pad may be at a comfortable temperature for a thirty-minute treatment, but the heat can build up over a long period and increase the chances of burning yourself.

If you're going to apply heat to your foot while you're in bed, do it with a hot water bottle which has the advantage of cooling off as your feet heat up.

Contrast Baths
Alternating hot and cold soaks is a great way to stimulate circulation. First soak your feet in warm water (98 to 102 degrees) for four minutes; then soak them in cool water (65 to 75 degrees) for one minute. Repeat four times, ending with the cold water.

This process exercises your blood vessels, making them alternately contract and relax, and increases your blood flow.

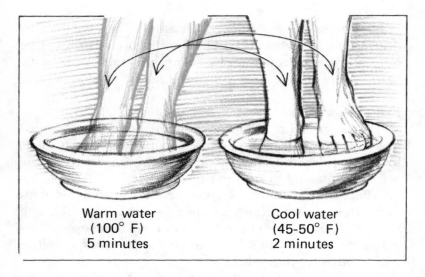

Warm water
(100° F)
5 minutes

Cool water
(45-50° F)
2 minutes

Soaking feet alternately in hot and cold water improves circulation.

If you have a circulation problem, this is great therapy to work into your daily routine.

Paraffin Baths

Another method of applying heat your doctor might prescribe is a paraffin bath. It's not a safe method to try at home and should be done, if at all, by a professional.

It is used to treat arthritis of the hands and feet and consists of applying a paraffin and mineral oil mixture to the foot. Enough mineral oil is added to the paraffin so that it reaches a melting point of 126 degrees, the temperature at which it is applied to your skin.

Paraffin baths should be avoided if you have a severe circulatory problem affecting your foot.

OTHER TREATMENTS

Other professionally administered heat treatments include infrared light from a heat lamp and deep heat treatments using ultrasound. Ultrasound is the application of sound waves with frequencies too high to be audible. The waves stimulate your tissues, producing heat. It's one of the most potent deep tissue physical therapies. Ultrasound should not be used over fracture sites, metallic implants or electric devices such as cardiac pacemakers.

Ultraviolet Rays
Ultraviolet light can be used to kill bacteria and fungus when you have a severe infection. It can also be used to stimulate tissue repair, especially in infections like chronic ulcers. It is sometimes used to treat psoriasis.

Massage
Massage is great for stimulating circulation and helping old injuries heal. You can massage your own feet if you can reach them or you can have a friend massage them for you. Massage should be gentle, especially if your skin is dry and sensitive. Use a soothing lotion.

Counterirritation
Counterirritation is based on the principle that if you introduce a new pain or another intense sensation, it will block out the old pain.

Heat-producing ointments work on this principle. They increase the blood supply to the skin by irritating it. The increased blood supply usually dulls the sensation of pain. Ointments, massage and ultraviolet rays can be used as counterirritants. Suction cups are used, more commonly in Europe than in this country, as are acupuncture and electrical stimulation.

Electrical Stimulation

When you can't contract or exercise a muscle voluntarily, electric currents can be used to exercise it even when it is too sore to touch or massage.

The sensation is odd. You aren't moving the muscle and you don't feel anything stimulating it, but it's contracting and twitching beyond your control. Electrical stimulation can be used to exercise muscles that can't be moved. It can relieve pain and stimulate circulation, even for an immobilized part such as a leg in a cast.

Most of these physical therapy techniques should be performed by your podiatrist or by a licensed physical therapist. You can always massage your own feet at home, and it's usually safe to properly soak or ice a traumatized foot. Exercise is still the most effective home therapy if you're able to do it. Walking does all the things the other therapies described are designed to do. As your muscles contract and relax, they massage the inside of your foot, stimulate circulation and produce heat, often relieving pain, at least temporarily. The most important function of exercise is probably to stimulate circulation. Nothing is as important to healing as adequate blood flow.

ALTERNATIVE TREATMENTS

18

Who shall decide when doctors disagree?
—*Alexander Pope,* Moral Essays. Epistle III To Lord
Bathurst, *1732*

Some interesting inroads have been made in the areas of
other than traditional medicine. Long considered quack-
ery in this country, traditional Chinese acupuncture, for
example, is now used with impressive results in main-
stream medical establishments like the UCLA Pain Center.
This chapter is a brief introduction to three alternative
forms of therapy. These forms of alternative treatments
are usually controversial, and are presented here, without
specific recommendations, to help those who may benefit
from them.

If you'd like to know more, ask your local librarian to recommend reading materials. If you decide you'd like to try any of these, be sure to get a referral from a doctor you trust as you would in seeking any form of physical therapy.

REFLEXOLOGY

Ancient Asian teachings claim the feet are maps of our physical state. In the days before shoes, they say, feet were massaged as they walked on stones and uneven terrain that stimulated circulation and dispersed waste material that had settled in the lower extremities.

Like acupuncture, foot reflexology is based on reflex points that correspond to various organs and glands. If the tips of your toes are tender, for example, the problem could be either tight shoes or infected sinuses.

Reflexologists say massage doesn't cure physical ailments, but stimulating the nerve endings in the foot relieves tension in the corresponding body part. It helps break up deposits of chemical wastes in the foot and stimulates the body's own natural healing process.

Even the most orthodox doctors agree that massage stimulates circulation to a specific area and that good circulation is essential to the healing process.

If you want to try massaging your feet, make yourself comfortable. A good massage can take as long as an hour. First examine your soles for irritations or sores to avoid. Then start at the area just under the ball of your foot and rub along your second metatarsal in a rolling, circular motion. Now, massage each toe carefully, and slowly knead the sole of your foot, working small areas and moving up and down until you've covered the entire foot.

The more pressure you use and the more massages you do, the greater the results are said to be.

ACUPUNCTURE

Limited acupuncture is the insertion of a series of very thin, stainless steel needles into the skin at specific pressure points often located in the feet and lower legs which are thought to be maps of the organs. Acupuncture has been shown to stimulate the release of endorphins, morphine-like substances the brain produces to stifle pain. This finding was bolstered by the discovery that naloxone, a drug that counteracts the effects of morphine, also reverses the pain-relieving effects of acupuncture.

Acupuncturists seek to treat the mind and body as related parts of one system. They try to discover the problem underlying pain or a particular ailment and they try to eliminate any immediate discomfort.

Usually the insertion of the needles is painless and the more relaxed you are, the less likely you'll be to feel anything.

The traditional theory is that the life force fuels the body and normally travels through the 12 channels or meridians that run the length of it. Illness occurs when the flow is obstructed. Needles applied to corresponding pressure points release energy until balance is restored.

SHIATSU AND ACUPRESSURE

Shiatsu is a Japanese word meaning *finger pressure*. The principle is the same as in acupuncture but pressure points are manipulated with the thumbs rather than with needles.

As in acupuncture and reflexology, the sole is the mirror of your anatomy. The toes correspond to the head, eyes, ears and nose, the ball of the foot to the liver, gall bladder and pancreas, the longitudinal arch to the kidneys and small intestines and the heel to the sex organs. Excessive pain in any part of the foot is said to indicate a problem in the related part of the body.

Only a shiatsu practitioner can do complicated massages, but you can rejuvenate tired feet at home. Sit on a chair and rest your feet on the floor. The points you will massage (always pressing with the ball of the thumb, not the tip, for five to seven seconds) are along the recesses in the top of the foot between the long tendons.

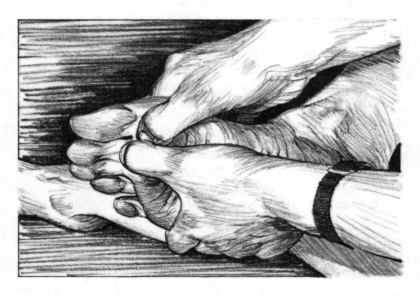

Simple massage helps soothe feet. Press with the ball of the thumb between tendons.

Place your thumbs behind the web space formed by the first two toes of the foot you're working on. Press for three seconds and pause. Moving from the middle of the foot toward the toes, repeat for three seconds and pause again. Repeat in each of the other three depressions between the tendons of your foot.

Cross your right leg over your left and grab your right big toe with your left thumb on top and your index finger underneath. Squeeze it for three seconds. Repeat at the joint and finally squeeze the toe from both sides.

Self-shiatsu is based on the idea that touch cannot only relieve specific problems but can also give you a generally wonderful sense of well-being. If pain is produced you should seek professional advice.

19

INSURANCE: ARE YOUR FEET COVERED?

*We can't cross a bridge until we come to it; but I
always like to lay down a pontoon ahead of time.*
—Bernard M. Baruch

When even simple surgery in your doctor's office can wipe
out a month's income and a week in the hospital costs as
much as a new car, the first questions about any form of
health care are: how much does it cost and does my
insurance cover it?

MEDICARE

If you're over 65 and collecting Social Security benefits or
if you're under 65 and have been collecting Social Security
disability benefits or have kidney disease referred to as
end-stage renal disease (ESRD) for at least two years,
you're eligible for Medicare. Social Security recipients are
automatically eligible for Part A, the hospital insurance

part, of Medicare that covers medically necessary hospital care and certain kinds of care following hospitalization. But Part B of Medicare, the Supplemental Medical Insurance (SMI), which covers doctor bills and a wide variety of other medical expenses, is voluntary. Such coverage, though, represents an excellent value because SMI is funded largely by federal general revenues. The SMI premium is deducted from your monthly benefit checks.

There are separate in-hospital (Part A) and outpatient (Part B) deductibles. (A deductible is the share of hospital and medical expenses which you must pay before your insurance policy starts paying.) After you've met the Part B deductible, Medicare pays 80 percent of the "reasonable charges" for covered services. The Medicare carrier in each area of the country determines the "reasonable charges" for covered services by reviewing actual charges made by the rendering practitioner and by all practitioners in the area during the previous year for the same procedure or service.

Medicare does cover surgery and other types of "medically necessary" foot care. Routine foot care like corn, callus and wart removal, treatment of flat feet and other structural problems and hygienic care is covered only if it is required treatment for a serious medical condition like diabetes or arteriosclerosis that affects the lower limbs.

On the other hand, Medicare guidelines are rather vague and it's best to check with your doctor and/or your local Medicare carrier about coverage for specific procedures.

There are two methods of getting Medicare payment of your Part B bills, and it's generally up to your doctor to decide which method to use. Try to persuade your doctor to use the "assignment method."

If your doctor agrees to the assignment method, he or she bills Medicare directly. By doing this your doctor is agreeing to accept Medicare's "reasonable charge" as full payment for his or her services. Medicare pays your doctor 80 percent of the reasonable charge minus any part of the deductible you haven't met. Your doctor then bills you for the remaining 20 percent plus any part of the deductible you haven't paid.

Under the "direct payment method," your doctor bills you or often requests payment at the time of your visit. Under this method there is no limit to what your doctor can charge. You then send a *Request for Payment* (or a claim) form with all the requested information to your local Medicare carrier. Medicare (the carrier) will in turn send you a check for 80 percent of the "reasonable charge" minus any outstanding portion of your Part B deductible. Your doctor or your local Social Security office can give you a form.

Be sure your doctor gives you a fully itemized bill or fills out all the appropriate items on the claim form, including a diagnosis of your problem. If you run into problems filling out the form, call your local Social Security office for assistance.

MEDICAID

If you are collecting welfare benefits such as Supplemental Security Income (SSI), you're probably eligible for Medicaid, a federal program administered by the states. Foot care by a licensed M.D. or podiatrist is generally covered under Medicaid. Fees for specific services are set in advance and the doctor is reimbursed by the state.

Some doctors won't accept Medicaid patients because they view the fee schedules as inadequate or are displeased with the time it takes to be reimbursed. Because coverage varies somewhat from state to state, you should check with your local Medicaid office or with your doctor about specific coverage. Eligibility for benefits is also determined by each state Medicaid program.

PRIVATE INSURANCE

Private insurance plans range from prepaid health maintenance organization (HMOs) that cover everything from office to hospital visits (some plans provide care at a clinic or hospital; others have you choose from a list of local doctors) to major medical coverage that protects you from the catastrophic expenses of a lengthy illness.

Because there are so many types of private health plans, it is difficult to generalize about foot care coverage.

For specific information you should check with your personnel office (if you're covered at work) or directly with your insurance carrier.

Questions to ask your insurer include:

What types of foot care are covered and what types are excluded under your policy?

What is the deductible? (A deductible is the share of the hospital and medical expenses you must pay before the insurance company starts paying.)

Does your plan cover the full cost of treatment or does it cover only a specific dollar amount set in advance that may not equal your doctor's fee?

Are benefits payable ("assignable") directly to your

doctor or to the hospital, or are you expected to pay and seek reimbursement?

Questions to ask your doctor include:

Does your doctor agree to bill the insurance company directly or does he or she expect you to pay for your treatment at the time services are rendered, requiring you to subsequently seek reimbursement from your insurance carrier?

Does your doctor agree to accept payment from your insurance company as payment in full?

Whatever coverage you have, the important thing is to understand what it will do for you and how it works. If you examine the benefits and limitations of your policy when you're healthy, you won't be taken by surprise when you're least interested in surprises—when you're sick or injured and need immediate medical care.

GLOSSARY

achilles tendon   the large tendon in the back of the ankle

ambulatory surgery   foot surgery performed in your doctor's office under local anesthesia after which you can usually walk away

analgesic   pain reliever

arteriosclerosis   thickening, hardening and loss of elasticity of the walls of blood vessels, especially arteries; commonly called hardening of the arteries

arthritis   inflammation of a joint; there are many types of arthritis with many causes; *see also* gout, osteoarthritis, rheumatoid arthritis

athlete's foot   a non-medical term used to describe fungus infections; fungus infections occur not only between the toes, on the sole of the foot and under the nails, but also on other parts of the body

ball of the foot   the front part of the foot, not including the toes; it is known more accurately as the metatarsal area

bedsores   ulcers that occur on the feet and other parts of the body when the victim is confined to bed and the prolonged pressure impairs circulation to the affected tissue

biomechanics   the study of the biology of motion and mechanics of motion

bunion   an inflammation around the joint where the big toe meets the first metatarsal; as the joint becomes increasingly deformed, the other toes are also pushed out of position

bursa   fluid-filled sac located over a joint and in other parts of the body to prevent excessive friction

bursitis   inflammation of a bursa

callus   a thickening of the skin developing from recurring friction and pressure

core calluses   a callus with a hard center or core

corn   a circumscribed, cone-shaped thickening of the skin, that develops because of recurrent friction and pressure

diabetes   a chronic, systemic disease marked by the secretion of excessive amounts of urine; diabetes mellitus, the most common form, is a metabolic disorder usually due to a malfunctioning pancreas causing high blood sugar

diabetic ulcer   an ulcer that appears on a diabetic person, usually at the site of an injury; it heals very slowly, if at all

edema   swelling; the presence of excessive fluid in the tissues

fallen arch   the lowering of the long arch between the heel and the big toe in which the foot turns outward and the weight of the body is taken up by the arch instead of by the toes and heel

fascia   a sheet or band of fibrous tissue

fat pad   a layer of fat that cushions the bottom of the foot

fissure   any crack, cleft or groove, normal or otherwise, in the skin of the foot—usually the heel

fungus nail a common nail problem resulting from the growth of fungus under the nail and characterized initially by dirty-looking yellow streaks along the nail

gout a form of arthritis caused by excessive uric acid in the blood that settles and crystallizes around the joints, particularly the joint of the big toe

hallux valgus a turning inward of the big toe that often causes bunions or other painful problems in the joint

hammertoe a toe deformed in a flexed position; since the toe is bent upward, the shoe often irritates it causing corns

heel counter the hard portion at the back of a shoe which cups the heel of the foot; the counter should be made of leather or plastic and not cardboard as in some inexpensive shoes

heel cup a device which cushions the bottom of the heel and can be used to cushion painful heel spurs

heel spur an edge or spur of bone that juts out of the heel bone and causes a great deal of pain

hematoma a swelling containing blood

hypertrophy excessive growth of a body part as in thickened nails

incurving nails nails that curve and grow directly into the skin; also called c-shaped nails

ingrown nail a nail that breaks through the adjacent skin and often becomes infected

intermittent claudication painful cramping of leg muscles that occurs with exercise but is relieved by rest; usually a symptom of a circulatory problem

ligament a band of strong fibers connecting one bone to another

lip of the nail adjacent skin on the sides of the nail

longitudinal arch   the area extending from the heel to the ball on the inner side of the foot

lymph   a pale fluid produced by the lymph glands; it contains white blood cells to fight infections

matrix of the nail   the area from which the nail grows

metatarsal   one of the long bones of the foot

metatarsal area   the area at the ball of the foot where the front ends of the metatarsal bones are found

microtrauma   very small trauma or wound; tearing

moleskin   a thick felt usually applied to protect the skin; it is available over-the-counter in most drugstores

nail bed   the skin under the nail

neuroma   thickened nerve tissue caused by chronic pressure on the nerve

orthosis   a custom-made device that conforms to an individual foot to help control motion, provide support, correct alignment or prevent or correct deformities

osteoarthritis   a form of arthritis caused by constant wear and tear on the joints; degenerative arthritis

osteoporosis   a potentially disabling condition in which the calcium content of the bones is depleted

plantar calluses   calluses on the sole or plantar area of the foot

plantar fascia   the tendon that connects the heel to the toes and runs along the arch of the foot

plantar fasciitis   inflammation of the plantar fascia

pump bump   a heel spur that occurs where the achilles tendon connects with the heel

pustule   a small elevation of the skin resembling a blister or pimple and containing pus, usually caused by excessive friction or pressure

rheumatoid arthritis   a chronic, systemic form of
arthritis characterized by recurring attacks of painful
joint inflammation; rheumatoid arthritis can become
progressively more acute over time but it can often be
controlled with medication

shank of a shoe   the sloping part of the shoe that
conforms to the bottom of the foot under the arch

soft corn   a corn found between the toes where
moisture keeps it soft; often caused by bony
protruberances of adjacent toes

sole   bottom of the foot

sole of a shoe   the part of the shoe covering the bottom
of the foot

sprain   a violent twisting, straining or pulling of a
ligament

stasis ulcer   ulcer caused by poor circulation; without
adequate circulation, the skin tends to break down
forming ulcerations

steroids   hormones usually injected to relieve swelling
and pain

stone bruise   bruised heel bone

strain   the pulling or twisting of a muscle or tendon

tendon   bands of strong fibers connecting muscle to
bone or to other parts, such as another tendon

toe box   the part of a shoe housing the toes

ulcer   a break in the continuity of tissue; often leads to
the disintegration of the underlying tissue

ultrasound   a form of physical therapy which uses deep
vibrations of sound waves to break up scar tissue,
increase circulation and decrease inflammation

upper   the part of a shoe or boot above the sole

varicose veins   abnormally swollen or enlarged veins

wart   a benign tumor, sometimes caused by a virus

INDEX

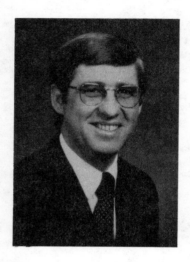

ABOUT THE AUTHORS

Timothy P. Shea, D.P.M., is the Consulting Podiatrist on the "Over Easy" television program.

He is active on the staffs of Mt. Diablo Hospital, John Muir Hospital and California College of Podiatric Medicine Hospital.

Dr. Shea is Clinical Professor, Department of Ambulatory Medicine, University of California Medical Center. He is also Associate Professor and Clinical Instructor, California College of Podiatric Medicine, San Francisco.

In addition, Dr. Shea is a Fellow, American College of Foot Orthopedists and Fellow, American Society for Laser Medicine and Surgery. He is board certified by the American Board of Podiatric Surgery.

Joan Smith is a journalist who lives in Mill Valley, California.

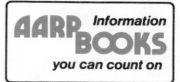

continued from other side

it contains many helpful suggestions for readers of all ages. Should be read by anyone who needs insurance. $5.95

It's Your Choice: The Practical Guide to Planning a Funeral provides guidance to both survivors arranging funerals for deceased loved ones, and to individuals formulating their own personal plans. This book *reveals key facts* about funeral prices, *legal requirements,* and *possible alternatives.* $4.95

Essential Guide to Wills, Estates, Trusts, and Death Taxes is designed to help you compose a will and plan an estate. Utilizing a question and answer format, this book unravels the mysteries of estate

planning with *simple, easily-understood information* and *level-headed advice.* $12.95

The Over Easy Foot Care Book $6.95

Name

Address

City/State   Zip

Send your order today to:
AARP Books
400 South Edward Street
Mount Prospect, IL 60056

Please add $1.30 shipping and handling per order. All orders must be prepaid.